Milk Supply

Edited by
Kathleen Kendall-Tackett, PhD, IBCLC, FAPA
& Scott Sherwood, BS

All royalties go to the
U.S. Lactation Consultant Association.

Praeclarus Press, LLC
©2015. United States Lactation Consultant Association

Praeclarus Press, LLC

2504 Sweetgum Lane

Amarillo, Texas 79124 USA

806-367-9950

www.PraeclarusPress.com

DISCLAIMER

The information contained in this publication is advisory only and is not intended to replace sound clinical judgment or individualized patient care. The author disclaims all warranties, whether expressed or implied, including any warranty as the quality, accuracy, safety, or suitability of this information for any particular purpose.

ISBN #978-1-939807-34-2

Cover Design: Ken Tackett

Acquisition & Development: Kathleen Kendall-Tackett & Scott Sherwood

Copy Editing: Kathleen Kendall-Tackett

Layout & Design: Nelly Murariu

Operations: Scott Sherwood

Contents

USLCA

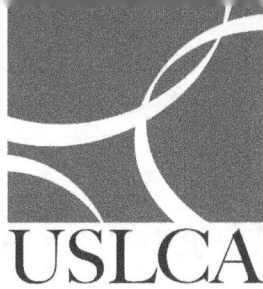

The Magic Number and Long-Term Milk Production

Nancy Mohrbacher, IBCLC, RLC, FILCA[1]

Keywords: Milk production, breast expressions, pumping, breastfeeding goals

Worry about milk production is the most common reason women wean earlier than planned. In many cases this worry is due to confusion about how milk production works. This article describes a teaching concept, termed the Magic Number. Clinicians can use this concept to provide mothers who are not exclusively breastfeeding on cue a clear, evidence-based understanding of how to keep their milk production stable over the long term.

With unrestricted access to the breast, most babies can easily adjust their mother's milk production by simply changing their breastfeeding length and frequency. However, many mothers with milk-production issues are not exclusively breastfeeding. Employed mothers,

---

1   nancymohrbacher@gmail.com

exclusively pumping mothers, and mothers using feeding schedules often seek help from clinicians when their milk production slows. Or they may ask for help in preventing milk production from slowing over the long term.

When milk production is not regulated solely by the baby, one teaching concept used successfully is the Magic Number (Mohrbacher, 2010). This term refers to the number of times each day a mother needs to remove milk from her breasts to maintain her milk production. If her number of daily milk removals stays at or above this threshold, her milk production stays steady or may even increase. If it falls below this threshold, her milk production slows.

Two Major Dynamics Determine a Mother's Magic Number
- Breast fullness
- Breast storage capacity

This specific threshold varies among mothers. Two primary dynamics determine an individual mother's Magic Number: degree of breast fullness and breast storage capacity. The purpose of this teaching concept is to give mothers a clear understanding of these dynamics and take the mystery and anxiety out of milk production. This knowledge, when provided with several other key facts, enhances mothers' confidence in breastfeeding and empowers them to adjust their daily routine as needed to meet their long-term goals.

Degree of Breast Fullness

Mothers are sometimes told to wait until their breasts feel full before expressing or breastfeeding. This advice reflects a basic misunderstanding of how milk production works. Research has found that the fuller breasts become, the more milk production slows (Kent, 2007).

One simple way to explain this mechanism to mothers is: full breasts make milk slower (Mohrbacher & Kendall-Tackett, 2010).

The opposite is also true. Milk production speeds when a mother's breasts are drained more fully. This is how a baby adjusts his mother's milk production as needed. If a baby wants more milk, he breastfeeds more often and/or longer. Taking a larger percentage of the available milk speeds the rate of milk production. In other words, drained breasts make milk faster.

Within a day, and even from feeding to feeding, rate of milk production can change dramatically. In one study, for example, after 6 hours without milk removal, one mother's rate of milk production per breast was 22 mL (about 2/3 oz.) per hour (Daly, Kent, Owens, & Hartmann, 1996).

By breastfeeding from that breast every 90 minutes and removing milk from her breasts more completely, her rate of production per breast increased quickly within the same day to 56 mL (nearly 2 oz.) per hour—more than double the previous rate.

Breast Storage Capacity

A mother's breast storage capacity refers to the maximum volume of milk available to her baby when her breast is at its fullest. Unrelated to breast size, breast storage capacity is determined by the amount of room in her milk-making glandular tissue. Breast size is determined primarily by the amount of fatty tissue (Geddes, 2007).

The maximum volume of milk in the breasts each day can vary greatly among mothers. Two studies found a breast storage capacity range among its mothers of 74 to 606 g (2.6 to 20.5 oz.) per breast (Daly, Owens, & Hartmann, 1993; Kent et al., 2006). The mother with the largest breast storage capacity accumulated up to 90% of her baby's daily milk intake in both breasts, while the one with the smallest storage capacity accumulated in both breasts only 20% of her baby's daily milk intake.

Breast storage capacity affects how long it takes for mother's breast to become full. For example, a woman with a small storage capacity may become so full with 2.5 ounces (75 mL) of milk in her breasts that her rate of milk production slows. However, in a woman with a larger breast storage capacity this same 2.5 ounces (75 mL) would not cause milk production to slow. This larger-capacity mother could, therefore, go for longer periods between feedings without her rate of milk production slowing.

It's vital to note that although breast storage capacity can affect feeding patterns, it does not affect a mother's overall ability to produce ample milk for her baby. One study found that all of its babies whose mothers had a small storage capacity had healthy weight gains (Kent et al., 2006). To consume the same amount of milk as other babies, however, on average these babies breastfed more times each day.

Depending on her breast storage capacity, a mother's Magic Number (number of daily milk removals needed to keep milk production stable) may be as few as 3, 4, or 5 or as many as 10, 11, or 12. But when a mother's total number of milk removals (breastfeedings plus milk expressions) dips below her Magic Number, her rate of milk production slows.

Facts and Focus

In addition to understanding degree of breast fullness and breast storage capacity, there is one key fact that is helpful for these mothers to know. Most employed and exclusively pumping mothers think that as their baby grows bigger and heavier they will need to increase their milk production.

They assume that—like babies fed formula—their breastfed babies will need more and more milk as they grow. These mothers are usually tremendously relieved to learn that the amount of milk breastfed babies consume daily between 1 and 6 months of age stays remarkably stable, on average between 25 and 30 oz. (750-900 mL), with an average increase during this time of only about 4 ounces (120 mL) or so (Butte, Lopez-Alarcon, & Garza, 2002). This means that when breastfeeding is going normally, after 1 month milk production doesn't need to increase by much. After reaching this level, a mother can focus primarily on maintenance until 6 months, when her baby's milk intake will decrease with the introduction of solid foods (Islam, Peerson, Ahmed, Dewey, & Brown, 2006).

To give mothers a clearer sense of how their daily choices affect their rate of milk production, it can be helpful to suggest employed mothers keep their focus on the 24-hour-day as a whole. By considering their baby's overall daily milk needs, it quickly becomes obvious that the more times each day the baby breastfeeds directly, the less expressed milk he will need while they're separated. In other words, every missed breastfeeding at home equals an average of 3 to 4 ounces (90-120 mL) more milk the baby needs while the mother is at work. Many mothers lose sight of the fact that encouraging babies to sleep more at night adds to the volume of expressed milk they need to leave during the day. Taking a broader view of their daily routine often provides the answers mothers need to maintain milk production over the long term.

As babies begin sleeping longer at night, number of milk removals can decrease. Also Western mothers are often encouraged to follow bottle-feeding norms by trying to convince their babies to take larger and less frequent feedings. This pattern, however, is not consistent with breastfeeding norms, as number of feedings per day have not been found to decrease between 1 and 6 months (Kent et al., 2006).

To stay aware of this dynamic, when an employed mother returns to work after maternity leave, at least once per week suggest she make note of how many times per day she removes milk from her breasts, adding breastfeedings and milk expressions. At least once per week, suggest exclusively pumping mothers total their daily milk yield. Milk production is easier to boost if it hasn't been reduced for longer than a couple of weeks. When a mother focuses weekly on either daily milk removals (employed mothers) or daily milk yield (exclusively pumping mothers), she will know when adjustments in routine are needed while it is still easy for her milk production to rebound.

Determining a Mother's Magic Number

An exclusively pumping mother will get an idea of her magic number quickly as she sees what level of daily milk expression maintains her milk production and when it starts to dip. Another clue to a mother's breast storage capacity, a major influencer of her Magic Number, is her milk yield at her first-morning expression.

In a 1996 survey of 10 exclusively pumping mothers, mothers who expressed 10 ounces (300 mL) of milk or more at the first-morning pumping were able to maintain their milk production long-term with as few as 5 milk expressions per day (Mohrbacher, 1996). Mothers who expressed 5 ounces (150 mL) or less at their first-morning pumping required more daily milk expressions to maintain milk production.

To get an idea of an employed mother's Magic Number (assuming she is exclusively breastfeeding a thriving baby), suggest she think back to her maternity leave. On average, how many times every 24 hours did her baby breastfeed? Because this daily number of feedings at the breast was working well for her baby, most likely this same number will keep her milk production stable.

So start with this daily total as an estimate of her Magic Number. For example, if her answer is 8 (which seems to be average), she can assume that to keep her milk production steady long term she will need to continue removing milk from her breasts at least 8 times each day. If she's expressing milk 3 times during her work day, this means she would need to breastfeed 5 times when she and her baby are together. Many employed mothers are diligent about maintaining their number of milk expressions at work. But often, as their baby gets older, they breastfeed less and less at home.

This change in routine can bring them below their Magic Number, slowing milk production. That's why it is important for a clinician not to limit her questions to the number of milk expressions at work.

Since milk production is determined by 24-hour milk-removal patterns, it is just as important to know about the breastfeeding routine at home. Another key piece of information is their longest stretch between milk removals (usually at night), which some mothers report may be as long as 12 hours.

Troubleshooting Using the Magic Number

One mother's experience provides a good example of how the Magic Number concept can be used. This mother called for help because she was expressing at work only about half of the milk her baby consumed at daycare and her goal was to breastfeed for at least a year. She was concerned that her milk was disappearing and that breastfeeding was at risk.

Her baby boy was 6 months old and she had returned to work 4 months earlier. She was away from her baby 5 days a week for 8 hours per day, including travel time. At work she expressed a total of 6 ounces (180 mL) of milk while her baby consumed 12 ounces (360 mL), which was near the average milk intake expected. When her volume of milk expressed at work began to decrease, this mother started taking galactogogues to increase her rate of milk production. While this would not be effective for every mother, it worked for her. However, every time she stopped taking the galactogogues, her milk production slowed again. She said that during her maternity leave, her baby had breastfed 9 times per day.

Now, though, her routine was very different:

» One breastfeeding at home before work

» Two milk expressions at work

» Two breastfeedings at home in the evening

» Baby was sleeping 10 to 12 hours at night as the longest stretch

Her total number of daily milk removals had dropped from 9 to 5 (3 breastfeedings at home plus 2 milk expressions at work).

The clinician gave this mother an explanation of how degree of breast fullness and breast storage capacity affects the Magic Number. The clinician concluded from the mother's description that the combination of her baby's 10-to-12-hour sleep stretch at night (full breasts make milk slower) and the drop in her total number of milk removals from 9 to 5, most likely explained her difficulty in maintaining her milk production.

When her baby started sleeping so long, at first the mother got up once during the night to express her milk, which allowed her to store enough milk for her workday. However, as her baby got older she stopped expressing at night and began breastfeeding fewer times at home, because her friends told her that older babies need fewer feedings.

After a better understanding of the dynamics affecting milk production, this mother realized that she her breast storage capacity was most likely near the small end of the spectrum. Now her experience made sense to her. Her goal was to breastfeed her baby for at least his first year, so she changed her daily routine. She started breastfeeding more often at home. She also decided that rather than waking her baby at night—which she most definitely did not want to do—she got up once during the night to express her milk. Armed with a clear understanding of how milk production worked, she knew how to adjust her daily routine so that she could meet her long-term breastfeeding goals. As a result, this mother had no more issues with her milk production and went on to meet her target goals.

The Magic Number is a teaching concept that focuses on the basics. Of course, in some cases a mother may have low milk-production for less common reasons, such as hypothyroidism, polycystic ovary syndrome (PCOS), the use of hormonal contraceptives, etc. Even so, it always makes sense to start with the fundamentals. Because milk production tends to be a very robust process, going back to basics is likely to address most mothers' milk-production issues. Over the millennia, the very survival of the human race has relied upon women's ability to produce milk. However, for an individual mother to meet her breastfeeding goals, first she needs to understand how this works.

Additional resources available online:

For employed mothers:

http://www.nancymohrbacher.com/blog/tag/for-employed-nursing-mothers

http://www.breastfeedingmadesimple.com/

For exclusively pumping mothers:

http://www.ameda.com/healthcare-professionals/videos/ameda-platinum-exclusive-pumping-video

References

Butte, N.F., Lopez-Alarcon, & Garza, C. (2002). *Nutrient adequacy of exclusive breastfeeding for the term infant during the first six months of life.* Geneva, Switzerland, World Health Organization. http://whqlibdoc. who.int/publications/9241562110.pdf

Daly, S. E., Kent, J. C., Owens, R. A., & Hartmann, P. E. (1996). Frequency and degree of milk removal and the short-term control of human milk synthesis. *Experimental Physiology, 81*(5), 861-875.

Daly, S. E., Owens, R. A., & Hartmann, P. E. (1993). The shortterm synthesis and infant-regulated removal of milk in lactating women. *Experimental Physiology, 78*(2), 209-220.

Geddes, D. T. (2007). Inside the lactating breast: The latest anatomy research. *Journal of Midwifery & Women's Health, 52*(6), 556-563.

Islam, M.M, Peerson, J.M., Ahmed, T., Dewey, K.G., & Brown, K.H. (2006). Effects of varied energy density of complementary goods on breast-milk intakes and total energy consumption by healthy,breastfed Bangladeshi children. *American Journal of Clinical Nutrition, 83*(4), 851-858.

Kent, J. C. (2007). How breastfeeding works. *Journal of Midwifery & Women's Health, 52*(6), 564-570.

Kent, J. C., Mitoulas, L. R., Cregan, M. D., Ramsay, D. T., Doherty, D. A., & Hartmann, P. E. (2006). Volume and frequency of breastfeedings and fat content of breast milk throughout the day. *Pediatrics, 117*(3), e387-395.

Mohrbacher, N. (1996). Mothers who forgo breastfeeding for pumping. *Circle of Caring, 9*(2), 1-2.

Mohrbacher, N. (2010). *Breastfeeding answers made simple: A guide for helping mothers.* Amarillo, TX: Hale Publishing.

Mohrbacher, N., & Kendall-Tackett, K. (2010). *Breastfeeding made simple: Seven natural laws for nursing mothers* (2nd Ed.). Oakland, CA: New Harbinger Publications.

Clinical Lactation, 2011, Vol. 2-1, 15-18

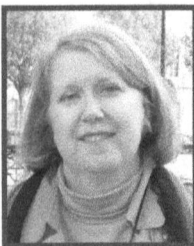

Nancy Mohrbacher, IBCLC, RLC, FILCA, is author of the books for breastfeeding specialists, *Breastfeeding Answers Made Simple (BAMS)* and *BAMS Pocket Guide Edition.* She is co-author (with Julie Stock) of all three editions of *The Breastfeeding Answer*

Book, a research-based counseling guide for lactation professionals, which has sold more than 130,000 copies worldwide. She is also co-author (with Kathleen Kendall-Tackett) of the popular book for parents, *Breastfeeding Made Simple: Seven Natural Laws for Nursing Mothers*. Her 2014 book, *Working and Breastfeeding Made Simple*, is available through Praeclarus Press. Nancy has written for many publications and speaks at events around the world. In 2008, the International Lactation Consultant Association officially recognized Nancy's contributions to the field of breastfeeding by awarding her the designation FILCA, Fellow of the International Lactation Consultant Association.

USLCA

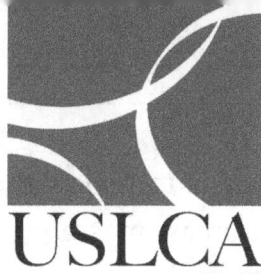

Breast Massage
A "Handy" Multipurpose Tool to Promote Breastfeeding Success

Betty Carlson Bowles, PhD, RNC, IBCLC, RLC[1]

Keywords: Breast massage, alternate breast massage, breast compression, hands-on pumping

Breast massage is not new. It is a "handy" technique that has been studied for decades and praised for its many uses in establishing and sustaining lactation, overcoming breast-feeding difficulties, and preventing or treating maternal and infant problems. This article reviews some of the studies examining various breast massage and breast-compression techniques, and proposes possible indications for their use.

One of the most powerful stimulants to the secretion of milk is massage of the breasts.

L. Emmett Holt, MD, 1899

For over a century there has been concern for early failure of breastfeeding, and attempts have been made to prevent the problems that precipitate that failure. The

1   betty.bowles@mwsu.edu

purpose of this article is to review the literature associated with the use of breast massage, and to summarize indications for its use.

Several mechanisms are believed to be responsible for the beneficial effects of breast massage on lactation. Because blood flow is closely correlated with the rate of milk secretion (Neville & Neifert, 1983), stimulating mammary blood flow with massage may enhance milk yield.

Massage and/or compression may mechanically move the milk out of the glands and ducts toward the nipple ensuring the subsequent production of milk. Various studies over the years have contributed to the evidence base related to breast massage.

Breast Massage Videos

Marmet

https://www.youtube.com/watch?v=Tuhuekl-3JY

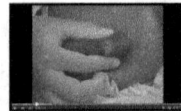

Morton & Colleagues

http://newborns.stanford.edu/Breastfeeding/HandExpression.html

http://newborns.stanford.edu/Breastfeeding/MaxProduction.html

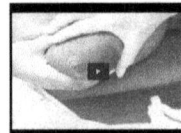

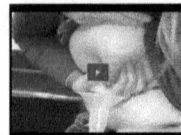

Newman & Kerneman

https://www.youtube.com/watch?v=Oh-nnTps1Ls

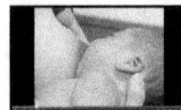

Waller (1946) identified engorgement as a leading cause of early breastfeeding failure. To prevent engorgement and subsequent pressure involution, he proposed the use of breast massage and manual expression.

Building on Waller's work, Iffrig (1967) used breast massage and putting the baby back to breast if the mother's breasts were still firm and tender after a feeding. This procedure resulted in softer, more comfortable breasts, and more satisfied babies.

The fact that many babies fell asleep before nursing again at both breasts led to the development of Alternate Breast Massage. This technique allows the baby to nurse while the mother observes the feeding pattern. When the nutritive sucking movements are long, slow, and rhythmic, accompanied by swallowing, the baby effectively removes milk and avoids production of sustained negative pressure that causes nipple injury.

Iffrig suggests when the sucking changes to a rapid and shallow non-nutritive sucking pattern followed by prolonged pauses, indicating slowed milk flow, the mother can start alternating breast massage with the baby's sucking.

With the baby still latched on, the mother gently massages the breast until the baby again sucks and swallows. She then suspends the massage until the baby resumes the non-nutritive sucking pattern. Thus the breast massage is alternated with the bursts of the baby's sucking. When one area softens she moves her fingers to a new position and continues alternating the massage with the baby's nursing until the entire breast has softened.

To study the effectiveness of Alternate Breast Massage, Iffrig (1968) took two groups of 30 mothers each: one group was taught the massage, and the other group was not taught the technique. The babies of mothers in both groups were weighed before and after feeding to determine the amount of milk ingested. Babies in the massage group consumed an average of 22.3 gm more per feeding than the babies in the non-massage group. When the daily totals were compared, the babies in the experimental group received an average of 4.5 ounces of milk more than the babies in the control group. Iffrig also observed that 97 of 100 mothers using the massage technique experienced neither painful breasts nor sore nipples. No control group was utilized in the latter phase of this study.

Inspired by the Iffrig study, Bowles, Stutte, and Hensley (1987/1988) recruited pregnant women from prenatal classes, which included a two-hour class on breastfeeding. Every other class was taught the Alternate Breast Massage technique. This resulted in 22 experimental and 29 control subjects. All babies were weighed at 4-to-6 week pediatric check-ups. Babies in the breast-massage group averaged weight gains of 10.33 gm/ day more than infants in the non-massage group, or nearly a pound more over the 4-to-6 week period. None of the mothers in the experimental group reported breast or nipple discomforts compared to 3% in the control group. Only 27% of mothers in the massage group expressed any concern for underproduction of milk compared to 59% of mothers in the control group.

Realizing that the breast was the research subject, not the mother or baby, Stutte, Bowles, and Morman (1988) had lactating women pump their breasts simultaneously using an electric breast pump, while massaging only one breast and utilizing the other breast as a control.

The procedure was repeated the following day with the women massaging the opposite breast. This resulted in 36 pairs of samples for comparison. Mean volume of milk pumped from the massaged breast was 4.8 ml greater than that from the nonmassaged breast. Mean creamatocrit from the massaged breast was 1.92% higher than from the non-massaged breast. These results indicate that breast massage can increase volume and fat content of breast milk. Increasing fat content coincidently increases caloric value.

Several researchers studied the effects of breast massage on hormone levels and breast-milk composition. Acknowledging that suckling is the most powerful stimulus for lactation, Yokoyama et al. (1994) compared the secretion of oxytocin and prolactin in response to suckling and breast massage. Six subjects received 20 minutes of their infant's suckling stimulus during breastfeeding, and six more received only breast massage and manual expression by a midwife. Blood samples for oxytocin and prolactin were drawn every two minutes from 10 minutes before the stimulus to the end of the stimulus period. In the suckling group, oxytocin was released in a pulsatile manner, but the difference in oxytocin level before and after suckling was low. In the breast-massage group, oxytocin levels stayed steady at high levels during the breast massage. Prolactin levels increased during sucking, but not during breast massage. In view of these findings, the authors recommend breast massage as an adjunct to infant suckling during breastfeeding.

Matthiesen et al. (2001) videotaped mother-infant dyads from birth through the first feeding and assessed infant hand movements and sucking behavior every 30 seconds. Blood samples were collected for oxytocin levels every 15 minutes. This study concluded that infants used their hands to explore and stimulate the breast in preparation for breastfeeding. A coordinated pattern was identified during nursing in which the infants alternated sucking and massage-like hand movements. Elevation in oxytocin levels followed periods of hand movements.

Foda, Kawashima, Nakamura, and colleagues (2004) took milk samples immediately before and after breast massage from healthy, exclusively breastfeeding mothers. Breast massage significantly increased total solids, lipids, casein concentration, and gross energy. Lactose was not significantly changed by breast massage.

Foda and Oku (2008) studied the effect of breast massage on breast-milk protein. Analyzing milk samples from 39 healthy breastfeeding mothers, they demonstrated a significantly increased whey protein concentration following breast massage.

Jones, Dimmock, and Spencer (2004) compared sequential and simultaneous breast pumping on volume and fat content of expressed milk, as well as the effect of breast massage on milk volume and fat content. Their results showed that simultaneous pumping is more effective in producing milk than sequential pumping, and that breast massage has an additive effect, improving milk expression by both methods.

The effect of breast massage on maternal comfort has also been studied. To test the effectiveness of preparation methods for breastfeeding, Storr (1987) studied 25 subjects who served as their own controls by preparing only one nipple and massaging one breast. Nipple tenderness and breast engorgement were assessed. Results indicated that tenderness and engorgement were decreased on the prepared and massaged breast. Examining the effects of alternative therapies to support breastfeeding, Ayers (2000) utilized breast massage consisting of moderate, even pressure to the breast from the base to areola by encompassing the breast with both hands and sliding them forward several times. This resulted in significantly less engorgement of the massaged breast.

Morton and colleagues (2009 a&b) described a hands-on pumping technique in which the mother used bilateral pumping with an electric breast pump while simultaneously compressing the breasts and massaging firmer areas. They demonstrated that pump-dependent mothers of preterm infants, and mothers otherwise at risk for insufficient milk production can attain and sustain good milk volumes using hands-on pumping and breast massage. They concluded that increased milk production results from more effective breast emptying rather than increasing the frequency or duration of the pumping sessions. They recommended that studies of pumping effectiveness should factor in the use of breast massage. Morton's video, *Hand Expression of Breastmilk*, demonstrates the use of gentle breast massage before hand expression to stimulate the flow of milk (Morton, 2009a). The video, *How to Use Your Hands When You Pump*, demonstrates the use of breast massage and compression during pumping to improve emptying of the breast to increase milk production. This technique emphasizes the importance of massaging the entire breast including the periphery (Morton, 2009b).

Descriptions of popular breast massage techniques can be found on the Internet. The Marmet Technique of manual expression recommends assisting the milk-ejection reflex by massaging the milk producing cells and ducts in a circular motion similar to that used in a breast examination (see link on p. 20). This massage technique is used in conjunction with light stroking motions from the base of the breast to the nipple and shaking the breast while leaning forward so gravity will help the milk eject (Marmet, 1999).

Newman and Kernerman (2008) propose that in the early weeks of life, infants tend to fall asleep when the milk flow slows, even if they have not had a good feeding. They describe a variation of Alternate Breast Massage, called Breast Compression, to continue the flow of milk when the baby pauses during nursing (see link on p. 20). This works especially well to assist the baby to get more colostrum in the early days of nursing.

Summary

Breast massage is not new. It is a *handy* technique that has been studied for decades and praised for its multiple uses for establishing and sustaining lactation, overcoming breastfeeding difficulties, and preventing or treating maternal and infant problems.

It can stimulate the milk-ejection reflex and improve the caloric content and volume of the milk supply. This may enable the mother to supplement her infant at the breast with her own breast milk, preventing unnecessary formula supplementation, and the premature weaning that inevitably results.

Other potential indications are listed in the accompanying table. However, the greatest benefit of this versatile, multipurpose technique is empowering the mother to respond to her own and her infant's needs, confident that through breastfeeding she is doing the very best for herself and her infant.

Clinical Lactation, 2011, Vol. 2-4, 21-24

Summary of Reasons to Try Breast Massage	
Goals	**Possible Indications**
To enhance normal breastfeeding:	All breastfeeding mother/baby dyads
To maximize colostrum intake to prevent:	Hypoglycemia Jaundice from delayed stooling
To promote efficient drainage/emptying of the breast during:	Engorgement Plugged ducts Mastitis Sore nipples
To establish and maintain the milk supply using a breast pump for:	Induced lactation/relactation Premature infants Gavage-fed infants Temporary suspension of breastfeeding due to breastmilk jaundice, maternal medication, hospitalization, etc.
To increase milk production and transfer for:	Failure to thrive Slow weight gain Growth spurts Sleepy infants Placid, *happy to starve* infants
To facilitate milk removal with minimal sucking effort for:	Sore nipples Craniofacial abnormalities Neurological defects Cardiorespiratory impairments
To maximize breastfeeding when there are negative effects from:	Hormonal contraception Smoking Supplementation Skipped feedings or baby sleeping all night Return to employment Nipple shield use Hemorrhage or anemia Retained placental fragments

References

Ayers, J.F. (2000). The use of alternative therapies in the support of breastfeeding. *Journal of Human Lactation, 16*(1), 52-56.

Bowles, B.C., Stutte, P.C., & Hensley, J.H. (December 1987/January 1988). New benefits from an old technique: Alternate massage in breastfeeding. *Genesis (ASPO/Lamaze), 9*(6), 5-9, 17.

Foda, M.I., Kawashima, T., Nakamura, S., Kobayashi, M., & Oku, T. (2004). Composition of milk obtained from unmassaged versus massaged breasts of lactating mothers. *Journal of Pediatric Gastroenterology and Nutrition, 38*, 484-487.

Foda, M.I., & Oku, T. (2008). Changes in milk protein of lactating mothers following breast massage. *International Journal of Dairy Science, 3*(2), 86-92.

Holt, L.E. (1899). *The diseases of infancy and childhood.* New York: D. Appleton and Company.

Iffrig, M.C. (1967). Early breastfeeding with alternate massage. *International Journal of Nursing Studies, 4*, 193-200.

Iffrig, M.C. (1968). Nursing care and success in breastfeeding. *Nursing Clinics of North America, 3*(2), 345-354.

Jones, E., Dimmock, P.W., & Spencer, S.A. (2004). A randomized controlled trial to compare methods of milk expression after preterm delivery. *Archives of Diseases of Children Fetal Neonatal Education, 85*, F91-F95.

Marmet, C. (1999). *Learn how to hand express breast milk.* Retrieved from http://www.ivillage.com/learn-how-hand-express-breastmilk/6-a-127422?p=2

Matthiesen, A.S., Ransjo-Arvidson, A.B., Nissen, E., & Uvnas-Moberg, K. (2001). Postpartum maternal oxytocin release by newborns: Effects of infant hand massage and sucking. *Birth, 28*(1), 13-19.

Morton, J., Hall, J.Y., Wong, R.J., Thairu, L., Benitz, W.E., & Rinne, W.D. (2009). Combining hand techniques with electric pumping increased milk production in mothers of preterm infants. *Journal of Perinatology, 29*, 757-764.

Morton, J. (2009a). *Hand expression of breast milk.* Retrieved from http://newborns.stanford.edu/Breastfeeding/HandExpression.html

Morton, J. (2009b). *Maximizing milk production with hands on pumping.* Retrieved from http://newborns.stanford.edu/Breastfeeding/MaxProduction.html

Neville, M.C., & Neifert, M.R. (1983). *Lactation: Physiology, nutrition, and breastfeeding*. New York: Plenum Press.

Newman, J., & Kernerman, E. (2008). *Breastfeeding help: Breast compression*. Retrieved from https://www.youtube.com/watch?v=ex5Var5urPU

Storr, G.B. (1987). Prevention of nipple tenderness and breast engorgement in the postpartal period. *Journal of Obstetric, Gynecologic, and Neonatal Nursing, 15*, 203-209.

Stutte, P.C., Bowles, B.C., & Morman, G.Y. (April/May 1988). The effects of breast massage on volume and fat content of human milk. *Genesis (ASPO/Lamaze), 10*(2), 22-25.

Waller, H. (1946). The early failure of breastfeeding. *Archives of Diseases of Childhood, 21*, 1-12.

Yokoyama, Y., Ueda, T., Irahara, M., & Aono, T. (1994). Releases of oxytocin and prolactin during breast massage and suckling in puerperal women. *European Journal of Obstetrics & Gynecology & Reproductive Biology, 53*, 17-20.

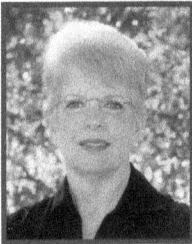

Betty Carlson Bowles, PhD, RNC, IBCLC, RLC, is Assistant Professor of Nursing at Midwestern State University in Wichita Falls, TX, teaching Nursing the Childbearing Family, Community Nursing and Pathophysiology. She is a Childbirth Educator and Lactation Consultant.

USLCA

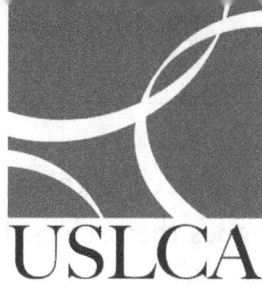

New Galactogogue Protocol, New Attitude?

Kathleen Marinelli, MD, IBCLC, RLC, FABM

Keywords: Galactogogues, milk supply, breastfeeding

In February, a new Academy of Breastfeeding Medicine (ABM) protocol was published in *Breastfeeding Medicine*: ABM Clinical Protocol #9: *Use of Galactogogues in Initiating or Augmenting the Rate of Maternal Milk Secretion* (First Revision January 2011). I am writing now having my hat on as ABM Protocol Committee Chair.

When we wrote the first version of this protocol in 2004, the basic message of the document was that galactagogues were a definite second-tier therapy for increasing milk supply, after all the mechanical and physical and otherwise treatable etiologies were investigated and adequately treated. That they are second-tier has not changed in this newest version.

What has subtly shifted is the attitude toward the use of the galactogogues themselves. In 2004, there was an almost *laissez-faire* attitude—if the mechanical changes and medical work-up did not yield the hoped-for increased results in milk production, then galactogogues were effective, and thus should be, and were, used. Although one should think (briefly) about potential side-effects, they were really quite rare, and the use of galactogogues were essentially standard of care (although not definitively stated as such). The protocol proceeded to tell us how to use them.

The 2011 revision gives us a different message. It is a prime example of why protocols need to be reviewed, and revised, with all the blood, sweat, and tears that involves for the primary contributors, and for so many of us, every 5 years. In this case, the careful searching out and evaluation of interim evidence-based studies and emerging information regarding more serious potential side effects of some galactogogues resulted in a shift in the ABM's recommendations regarding these drugs and herbs.

This newer data suggests that we should exercise more caution in recommending these drugs to induce or increase the rate of milk secretion in lactating women, particularly in women without specific risk factors for insufficient milk supply. There have been more significant side effects documented for some of them.

We are also now using Levels of Evidence when stating recommendations. The Levels of Evidence are based on the United States Preventive Services Task Force, *Quality of Evidence* (last accessed February 12, 2011).

Each study reviewed is classified by the authors according to these Levels, and when a recommendation is made in the protocol, we give the Level of Evidence so that the reader has an idea how strongly the recommendation can or should be taken (e.g., Level I is a randomized, controlled study). In this way, we feel we give you a better idea of the strength of the recommendation, based on the strength of the data behind it.

Consequently, as you read this revised protocol, you may be surprised to realize that the evidence for using pharmacologic and herbal galactagogues has grown weaker. There are still some clinical situations that appear to warrant their use. But there clearly also appears to be a knowledge gap, and yet another area ripe for research. Check out the new protocol, and let us know what you think.

Reprinted from the Academy of Breastfeeding Medicine blog, *February 11, 2011, with permission of the author and the Academy of Breastfeeding Medicine..*

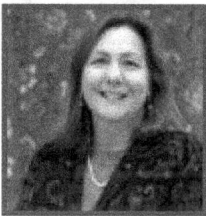

Kathleen Marinelli, MD, IBCLC, RLC, FABM, is an Associate Professor of Pediatrics and the University of Connecticut School of Medicine, and directs Lactation Support Services at Connecticut Children's Medical Center, Hartford, CT. She is chair of the U.S. Breastfeeding Committee, and serves as the Chair of the Protocol Committee for the Academy of Breastfeeding Medicine. Her research interests center on breastfeeding and the use of human milk and donor milk banking. She has lectured extensively in the U.S. and abroad.

USLCA

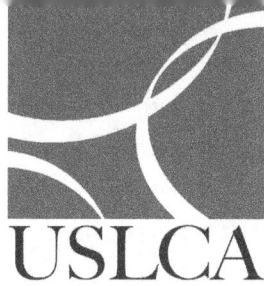

ABM Clinical Protocol #9: Use of Galactogogues in Initiating or Augmenting the Rate of Maternal Milk Secretion

(First Revision January 2011)

Breastfeeding Medicine Volume 6, Number 1, 2011

©Mary Ann Liebert, Inc. DOI:10.1089/bfm.2011.9998.

The Academy of Breastfeeding Medicine Protocol Committee

A central goal of The Academy of Breastfeeding Medicine is the development of clinical protocols for managing common medical problems that may impact breastfeeding success. These protocols serve only as guidelines for the care of breastfeeding mothers and infants and do not delineate an exclusive course of treatment or serve as standards of medical care. Variations in treatment may be appropriate according to the needs of an individual patient. These guidelines are not intended to be all-inclusive, but to provide a basic framework for physician education regarding breastfeeding.

Background

Galactogogues (or lactogogues) are medications or other substances believed to assist initiation, maintenance, or augmentation of the rate of maternal milk synthesis. Because perceived or actual low milk supply is one of the most common reasons given for discontinuing breast-feeding,[1-8] both mothers and health professionals have sought medication(s) to address this concern. Evaluation of evidence-based studies and emerging information regarding more serious potential side effects of some galactogogues have resulted in a recent shift in the Academy of Breastfeeding Medicine's recommendations regarding these drugs and herbs. In 2004, the previous version of this protocol used existing evidence that prescription galactogogues were effective and described when and how to use them.[9] Emerging data suggest that we should exercise more caution in recommending these drugs to induce or increase the rate of milk secretion in lactating women, particularly in women without specific risk factors for insufficient milk supply.

Human milk production is a complex physiologic process involving physical and emotional factors and the interaction of multiple hormones, the most important of which is believed to be prolactin. Despite the fact that prolactin is required for lactation, there has been no evidence for direct correlation of serum prolactin levels (baseline or percentage increase after suckling) with the volume of milk production in lactating women.[10–12]

Lactation is initiated with parturition, expulsion of the placenta, and falling progesterone levels in the presence of very high prolactin levels. Systemic endocrine control of other supporting hormones (estrogen, progesterone, oxytocin, growth hormone, glucocorticoids, and insulin) is also important.[13] These hormonal changes trigger secretory activation (lactogenesis II) of the mammary secretory epithelial cells, also called lactocytes. Prolactin secretion functions in a negative feedback system in which dopamine serves as an inhibitor. Therefore, when dopamine concentration decreases, prolactin secretion from the anterior pituitary increases. The theory behind pharmaceutical galactogogues is that dopamine antago-nists increase prolactin secretion[14] and subsequently increase the overall rate of milk synthesis. However, as mentioned above, no correlation exists between serum prolactin and increased milk volume.[10–12]

After secretory activation, the rate of milk synthesis is controlled locally in the mammary gland by autocrine control. Lactating breasts are never completely "empty" of milk, so the terms "drain, drainage, draining," etc., are more appropriate. If the breasts are not drained regularly and thoroughly, milk production declines. Alternatively, more frequent and thorough drainage of the breasts typically results in an increased rate of milk secretion, with both a rapid (per feeding) effect and a delayed (several days) effect.[12] Even though the rate of milk synthesis is controlled locally at this stage of lactation, suckling-induced peaks of prolactin continue throughout the entire course of breastfeeding.

Potential Indications for Galactogogues

Galactogogues commonly have been used to increase a faltering rate of milk production, often due to the effects of maternal or infant illness and hospitalization or because of regular separation such as work or school. One very common area of use has been the neonatal intensive care unit, where the aim has been to stimulate initial secretory activation or augment declining milk secretion in these mothers. Mothers who are not breastfeeding but are expressing milk by hand or with a pump often experience a decline in milk production after several weeks. Galactogogues have also been used for adoptive breastfeeding (induction of lactation in a woman who was not pregnant with the current child) and relactation (reestablishing milk secretion after weaning). Many breastfeeding medicine specialists and lactation consultants have recommended these drugs and herbs, usually as a last resort when other non-pharmacological measures have not resulted in an increase in milk volumes. However, some providers may inappropriately recommend galactogogues prior to emphasizing the primary means of increasing the overall rate of milk synthesis (i.e., frequent feeding and complete milk removal at regular intervals) or evaluating other medical factors that potentially may be involved.

Pharmaceutical Galactogogues

Currently available pharmaceutical galactogogues are all dopamine antagonists and will increase prolactin levels via this mechanism.[12] A number of older studies documented increased baseline prolactin levels in lactating women who took metoclopramide or domperidone.[15-20] However, there are only a few randomized, placebo-controlled, blinded studies on each of these agents, and these studies are small.

Domperidone

Regarding domperidone, there are two well-designed randomized, placebo-controlled, blinded studies. One of the studies, published in 2010 (n¼46), shows that domperidone is associated with significantly increased volumes of expressed milk among women with premature infants less than 31 weeks' gestation; the study concluded at 14 days, so longerterm effects cannot be evaluated.[11] One very small study (n¼6) suggests that individual women may be "responders" or "non-responders" and that primiparas may respond to domperidone with higher prolactin levels than multiparas."[21]

Metoclopramide

For metoclopramide, only four randomized, placebocontrolled, blinded studies have been published, and they each have some problem(s) in design, small sample size, and/ or patient selection.[22–25] Metoclopramide did not produce a statistically significant effect on infant weight gain in a randomized controlled trial of metoclopramide versus placebo in a 2008 study of 20 mothers who were relactating: 10 women received metoclopramide, and 10 received placebo; all received a course of standardized counseling regarding optimal breastfeeding technique.[24]

These results replicated an earlier study with a total of 50 mothers.25 All our of these higherquality studies[22–25] found no differences in milk volumes and/or duration of breastfeeding between etoclopramide and placebo. Two found optimal breastfeeding instruction or counseling to be positively associated with a statistically significant increase in infant weight gain (and corresponding decrease in use of supplemental feedings).[24,25] The other two did not evaluate or assist with optimal breastfeeding routines.[22,23]

Summary

Despite widespread use of these pharmaceutical galacto-gogues, there are important reasons for reconsideration of this practice:

» Galactogogues do increase baseline serum prolactin, but there is no direct correlation between baseline prolactin levels and rates of milk synthesis or measured volumes of milk production.

» Previous studies up through 2006 have tended to show a pattern of increased milk production, but they have generally been of poor quality,9,10 with the following weaknesses:

- Lack of randomization, controls, or blinding

- Small sample sizes

- High dropout rates

- Nonpharmacological measures were not optimized.

» Older reviews have cited studies with positive results while minimizing or ignoring studies with negative results. [9,26,27]

» A key systematic review in 2007[10] found two main problems.

- Evidence for the use of pharmaceutical galactogogues is lacking: Only seven studies of various galactogogues met evidence-based criteria for review.

- Potential significant side effects of the drugs should be weighed carefully against the lack of evidence (see Appendix for potential risks and benefits of specific drugs).

- Prescription drugs used as galactogogues constitute "off-label" use in most countries (they are not approved by regulatory agencies for this indication).

Herbals, Foods, and Beverages as Galactogogues

In non-Western cultures, postpartum women are assisted in a number of ways that are intended to ease their transition to motherhood and to optimize breastfeeding. Many cultures keep new mothers very warm and insist on a period of rest of approximately 1 month. Many also have traditional foods and herbs for postpartum women that are meant to increase the mother's strength and enhance lactation.[28]

Many of these herbal remedies have been used throughout history to enhance milk supply. Some herbs mentioned as galactogogues include fenugreek, goat's rue, milk thistle (Silybum marianum), oats, dandelion, millet, seaweed, anise, basil, blessed thistle, fennel seeds, marshmallow, and many others. Although beer is used in some cultures, alcohol may actually reduce milk production. A barley component of beer (even nonalcoholic beer) can increase prolactin secretion, but there are "no systematic studies" and "there is no hard evidence for causal effect."[29,30]

The mechanism(s) of action for most herbals are unknown. Most of them have not been scientifically evaluated, but traditional use suggests safety and possible efficacy. The available studies for herbs, herbal medicines, or herbal galactogogues suffer from the same deficiencies as the studies for pharmacologic agents: Small numbers of subjects, lack of information regarding breastfeeding advice, and lack of randomization, controls, or blinding

(Levels of Evidence II-1,31 II-332).[1] The placebo effect may be the reason for widespread impressions (anecdotal experience) of a positive effect of fenugreek on increased milk volumes (Level of Evidence III, personal communications from K.A. Marinelli [2010], N. Wight [2010], C. Smillie [2009], and N.G. Powers [2010]). The minimal specific data regarding these herbs are presented in the Appendix.

It is important to note that caution is required for the use of herbal preparations because of the lack of standardized dosing preparations (other than research settings), possible contaminants, allergic potential, and drug interactions. Several herbs, taken orally, will increase patient blood levels of warfarin, heparin, and other anticoagulants. There are several reports of severe maternal allergic reactions to fenugreek.[33]

Practice Recommendations

The following recommendations, based upon current evidence, apply to women experiencing difficulties with a low rate of milk production (e.g., the baby is not gaining weight normally or supplementation is being used because of low milk production, during either the initiation or maintenance of milk supply).

Specific information about individual drugs and herbs is summarized at the end of these recommendations in the Appendix.

---

1   Levels of Evidence are based on the United States Preventive Services Task Force "Quality of Evidence" (www.ncbi.nlm.nih.gov/books/NBK15430, last accessed December 20, 2010).

1. Evaluate and augment the frequency and thoroughness of milk removal. Use non-pharmacologic measures to increase the overall rate of breastmilk synthesis.

   a. For women with healthy term infants: Improve breastfeeding practices (Level of Evidence I).

      i. Recommend skin-to-skin contact between mother and baby to facilitate frequent feeding and stimulate oxytocin release (the milk ejection reflex [MER]).[34]

      ii. Encourage mother to perform self-breast massage in order to improve oxytocin release (MER) and milk removal.

      iii. Review or teach relaxation techniques to facilitate oxytocin release (MER) for improved milk removal.

      iv. Help the mother–infant dyad to achieve optimal latch-on.[10,24,25]

      v. Resolve nipple pain, if applicable, using the following strategies:

         (1) Optimal latch-on

         (2) Diagnosis and management of other causes of pain

         (3) Refer to a lactation specialist as needed.

      vi. Emphasize unrestricted frequency and duration of breastfeeding (if the infant has been shown to be effectively transferring milk).[24,25]

vii. Advise the mother to reduce or stop unnecessary supplementation35 and provide strategies for how to do so.

(1) Gradual tapering off of amounts of supplementation

(2) Use of "supplementer system" (tube at the breast attached to a source of supplemental milk) if appropriate.

b. For women with babies who are ineffective at milk removal or unable to feed at the breast (e.g., premature, hospitalized, hypotonic):

i. Recommend and teach gentle hand expression of colostrum: The volume extracted by hand expression is greater than the volume extracted by fullsize, automatic cycling breast pumps;36 video and photographic illustrations of hand expression are available at newborns. http://newborns.stanford.edu/Breastfeeding/[37] and www.breastfeeding.com/helpme/helpme_images_expression.html.[38]

ii. Recommend milk expression with a full-size, automatic cycling breast pump, capable of draining both breasts at the same time ("hospital grade"), if available (Level of Evidence II-2).[39]

iii. Recommend "hands-on pumping" (a combination of hand expression with double pumping); this technique was superior to double pumping alone in one randomized, controlled trial[40] and one observational study[41] (Level of Evidence I and II-3).

    iv. Recommend that women adjust the electric pump to their maximum comfortable vacuum, which enhances milk flow rate and milk yield and minimizes occurrence of tissue damage (Level of Evidence II-1).[42]

    v. Recommend hand expression if a hospital-grade pump is not available or if the woman prefers the manual technique; hand expression requires instruction and a period of practice until the mother becomes proficient.

    vi. Foot pump expression does not require electricity and may be another available alternative.[43]

2. Evaluate the mother for "medical" causes of hypogalactia: Pregnancy, medications, primary mammary glandular insufficiency, breast surgery, polycystic ovary syndrome, hypothyroidism, retained placenta, theca lutein cyst, loss of prolactin secretion following postpartum hemorrhage, heavy smoking or alcohol use, or other pertinent conditions. Treat the condition as indicated, if treatment is available[12] (Level of Evidence II-2, II-3, and III).

3. Because current research of all galactogogues is relatively inconclusive and all of the agents have potential adverse effects, ABM cannot recommend any specific pharmacologic or herbal galactogogues at this time.

4. The healthcare provider who weighs the potential risks versus the potential benefits of these agents and chooses to prescribe a galactogogue should follow the guidelines below (Level of Evidence III) (see Appendix regarding details of prescribing specific galactogogues).

5. Inform women about available data concerning efficacy, timing of use, and duration of therapy of galactogogues (Level of Evidence I).[10] (Specific information is presented in the Appendix.)

6. Inform women about available data concerning potential adverse effects of galactogogues (see Appendix regarding details of specific galactogogues):

   a. Screen the mother for allergies to, contraindications to, or drug interactions with the chosen medication or other substance.

   b. Provide ongoing care to, supervise ongoing care of, or transfer care of both mother and infant to ensure appropriate follow-up and attention to any side effects.

   c. Prescribe galactogogues at the lowest possible doses for the shortest period of time; do not exceed recommended therapeutic doses.

   d. Consider gradually discontinuing the drug (tapering the dose) at the end of therapy; some studies stop the drug at the conclusion of therapy, and others gradually discontinue the drug, with no clear advantage to either method.

e. If milk production wanes after stopping the drug and improves again with resumption of the medication, attempt to gradually decrease the drug to the lowest effective dose and then discontinue the drug at a later date if possible.

f. Consider obtaining written documentation of informed consent when using any galactogogues.

Conclusions

Prior to the use of a galactogogue, thorough evaluation should be performed of the entire feeding process by a lactation expert. Reassurance may be offered, if appropriate. When intervention is indicated for the dyad, modifiable factors should be addressed: comfort and relaxation for the mother, frequency and thoroughness of milk removal, and underlying medical conditions. Medication should never replace evaluation and counseling on modifiable factors.

As new evidence has emerged regarding various interventions to increase milk secretion in lactating women, the case for using pharmaceutical galactogogues has grown weaker. There remain selected indications for which some of these agents may be useful, but the data are insufficient to make definitive recommendations. One high-quality study has found domperidone useful in mothers of babies less than 31 weeks' gestation in the neonatal intensive care unit (see the Appendix). Herbal galactogogues are problematic because of lack of regulation of preparations and insufficient evidence of efficacy and safety. Clinicians should prescribe galactogogues with appropriate caution in regards to drug-to-drug (or drug-to-herb) interactions as well as an overall risk-to-benefit approach and complete informed consent. Close follow-up of both mother and baby is essential to monitor the status of lactation as well as any adverse effects of the drug(s) on mother or infant.

Recommendations for Further Research

Existing studies in this area cannot be considered conclusive, and many of the recommendations are based primarily on expert opinion, small studies, and studies in which nonpharmacologic breastfeeding support was suboptimal. Most studies have been done in mothers of preterm infants using mechanical breast pumps rather than in mothers of term infants whose problems usually arise in the first few days to weeks postpartum.

There is a clear need for well-designed, adequately powered, randomized, controlled trials using adequate doses of galactogogues in populations of women in which both the experimental and control groups receive modern, appropriate lactation support. These studies need to be done in mothers of both term and preterm infants and need to measure clinically relevant outcomes such as infant weight gain, need for artificial feeding (supplements other than mother's own milk), quantification of maternal milk synthesis, and adverse drug effects.

Acknowledgments

This work was supported in part by a grant from the Maternal and Child Health Bureau, U.S. Department of Health and Human Services.

References

1. Li R, Fein SB, Chen J, et al. Why mothers stop breastfeeding: Mothers' self-reported reasons for stopping during the first year. *Pediatrics* 2008;122(Suppl 2):S69–S76.

2. Dennis C, Hodnett E, Gallop R, et al. The effect of peer support on breast-feeding duration among primiparous women: A randomized controlled trial. *CMAJ* 2002;166:21–28.

3. Hauck YL, Fenwick J, Dhaliwal SS, et al. A Western Australian survey of breastfeeding initiation, prevalence and early cessation patterns. *Matern Child Health J* 2010 Jan 14 [Epub ahead of print]. www.springerlink.com/content/j462321682423568/ (accessed December 3, 2010).

4. Huang Y, Lee J, Huang C, et al. Factors related to maternal perception of milk supply while in the hospital. *J Nurs Res* 2009;17:179–188.

5. Lewis JA. Maternal perceptions of insufficient milk supply in breastfeeding. *Am J Matern Child Nurs* 2009;34:264.

6. McCann MF, Bender DE. Perceived insufficient milk as a barrier to optimal infant feeding: Examples from Bolivia. *J Biosoc Sci* 2006;38:341–364.

7. Otsuka K, Dennis C, Tatsuoka H, et al. The relationship between breastfeeding self-efficacy and perceived insufficient milk among Japanese mothers. *J Obstet Gynecol Neonatal Nurs* 2008;37:546–555.

8. Segura-Millan S, Dewey D, Perez-Escamilla R. Factors associated with perceived insufficient milk in a low-income urban population from Mexico. *J Nutr* 1994;124:202–212.

9. Academy of Breastfeeding Medicine. Use of Galactogogues in Initiating or Augmenting Maternal Milk Supply 2004. www.bfmed.org/Resources/Protocols.aspx (accessed December 3, 2010).

10. Anderson PO, Valdes V. A critical review of pharmaceutical galactogogues. *Breastfeed Med* 2007;2:229–242.

11. Campbell-Yeo ML, Allen AC, Joseph K, et al. Effect of domperidone on the composition of preterm human breast milk. *Pediatrics* 2010;125:e107–e114.

12. Lawrence RA, Lawrence RM. *Breastfeeding: A Guide for the Medical Profession*, 6th ed. Elsevier Mosby, Philadelphia, 2005.

13. Hale T, Hartmann P, eds. *Textbook of Human Lactation*. Hale Publishing, Amarillo, TX, 2007.

14. Murray L, ed. *Physicians' Desk Reference*, 63rd ed. Thomsen Reuters, Montvale, NJ, 2009.

15. Da Silva OP, Knoppert DC, Angelini MM, et al. Effect of domperidone on milk production in mothers of premature newborns: A randomized, double-blind, placebo-controlled trial. *CMAJ* 2001;164:17–21.

16. Ehrenkrantz RA, Ackerman BA. Metoclopramide effect on faltering milk production by mothers of premature infants. *Pediatrics* 1986;78:614–620.

17. Guzma'n V, Toscano G, Canales ES, et al. Improvement of defective lactation by using oral metoclopramide. *Acta Obstet Gynecol Scand* 1979;58:53–55.

18. Kauppila A, Anunti P, Kivinen S, et al. Metoclopramide and breast feeding: Efficacy and anterior pituitary responses of the mother and child. *Eur J Obstet Gynecol Reprod Biol* 1985;19:19–22.

19. Liu JH, Lee DW, Markoff E. Differential release of prolactin variants in postpartum and early follicular

20. Toppare MF, Laleli Y, Senses DA, et al. Metoclopramide for breast milk production. Nutr Res 1994;14:1019–1029.

21. Wan EWX, Davey K, Page-Sharp M, et al. Dose-effect study of domperidone as a galactagogue in preterm mothers with insufficient milk supply, and its transfer into milk. *Br J Clin Pharmacol* 2008;66:283–289.

22. Hansen WF, McAndrew S, Harris K, et al. Metoclopramide effect on breastfeeding the preterm infant: A randomized trial. *Obstet Gynecol* 2005;105:383–389.

23. Lewis PJ, Devenish C, Kahn C. Controlled trial of metoclopramide in the initiation of breast feeding. *Br J Clin Pharmacol* 1980;9:217–219.

24. Sakha K, Behbahan AG. Training for perfect breastfeeding or metoclopramide: Which one can promote lactation in nursing mothers? *Breastfeed Med* 2008;3:120–123.

25. Seema, Patwari AK, Satyanarayana L. An effective intervention to promote exclusive breastfeeding. *J Trop Pediatr* 1997;43:213–216.

26. Gabay MP. Galactogogues: Medications that induce lactation. *J Hum Lact* 2002;18:274–279.

27. Emery MM. Galactogogues: Drugs to induce lactation. *J Hum Lact* 1996;12:55–57.

28. Kim-Godwin YS. Postpartum beliefs and practices among non-Western cultures. *Am J Matern Child Nurs* 2003;28: 74–78.

29. Koletzko B, Lehner F. Beer and breastfeeding. *Adv Exp Med Biol* 2000;478:23–28.

30. Mennella JA, Beauchamp GK. Beer, breast feeding, and folklore. *Dev Psychobiol* 1993;26:459–466.

31. Di Pierro F, Callegari A, Carotenuto D, et al. Clinical efficacy, safety and tolerability of BIO-C® (micronized Silymarin) as a galactogogue. *Acta Biomed* 2008;79:205–210.

32. Swafford S, Berens P. Effect of fenugreek on breast milk volume [abstract]. *ABM News Views* 2000;6(3):21.

33. Tiran D. The use of fenugreek for breast feeding women. *Complement Ther Nurs Midwifery* 2003;9:155–156.

34. Uvnäs-Moberg K. *The Oxytocin Factor.* Perseus Books, Cambridge, MA, 2003.

35. Academy of Breastfeeding Medicine Protocol Committee. ABM Protocol #3: Hospital guidelines for the use of supplementary feedings in the healthy term breastfed neonate. Revised 2009. *Breastfeed Med* 2009;4:175–182.

36. Ohyama M, Watabe H, Hayasaka Y. Manual expression and electric breast pumping in the first 48 h after delivery. *Pediatr Int* 2010;52:39–43.

37. Morton J. Hand expression of breastmilk. http://newborns.stanford.edu/Breastfeeding/HandExpression.html (accessed December 3, 2010).

38. Breastfeeding.com. Expressing breastmilk. http://www.thebump.com/t/breastfeeding (accessed December 3, 2010).

39. Green D, Moye L, Schreiner RL, et al. The relative efficacy of four methods of human milk expression. *Early Hum Dev* 1982;6:153–159.

40. Jones E, Dimmock P, Spencer SA. A randomised controlled trial to compare methods of milk expression after preterm delivery. *Arch Dis Child Fetal Neonatal* 2001;85:F91–F95.

41. Morton J, Hall JY, Wong RJ, et al. Combining hand techniques with electric pumping increases milk production in mothers of preterm infants. *J Perinatol* 2009;29:757–764.

42. Kent JC, Mitoulas LR, Cregan MD, et al. Importance of vacuum for breastmilk expression. *Breastfeed Med* 2008;3:11–19.

43. Becker GE, McCormick FM, Renfrew MJ. Methods of milk expression for lactating women. *Cochrane Database Syst Rev* 2008;8(4):CD006170.

44. Rossi M, Giorgi G. Domperidone and long QT syndrome. *Curr Drug Saf* 2010;5:257–262.

45. Djeddi D, Kongolo G, Lefaix C, et al. Effect of domperidone on QT interval in neonates. *J Pediatr* 2008;153:663–666.

46. U.S. Food and Drug Administration. FDA Requires Boxed Warning and Risk Mitigation Strategy for Metoclopramide-Containing Drugs [news release February 26, 2009]. http://www.fda.gov/newsevents/newsroom/pressannouncements/ucm149533.htm (accessed December 3, 2010).

47. Gongadze N, Kezeli T, Antelava N. Prolong QT interval and "torsades de pointes" associated with different group of drugs. *Georgian Med News* 2007;153:45–49.

48. Pham CP, de Feiter PW, van der Kuy PH, et al. Long QTc interval and torsades de pointes caused by fluconazole. *Ann Pharmacother* 2006;40:1456–1461.

49. Domperidone and sudden death. *Prescrire Int* 2006;15:226.

50. Domperidone and sudden death. Cardiac rhythm disorders: QT interval prolongation. *Prescrire Int* 2008;17:67.

51. Collins KK, Sondheimer JM. Domperidone-induced QT prolongation: Add another drug to the list. *J Pediatr* 2008;153:596–598.

52. Straus SM, Sturkenboom MC, Bleumink GS, et al. Noncardiac QTc-prolonging drugs and the risk of sudden cardiac death. *Eur Heart J* 2005;26:2007–2012.

53. Jellin JM, Gregory PJ, Batz F, et al. *Natural Medicines Comprehensive Database.* Therapeutic Research Faculty, Stockton, CA, 2009.

54. Low Dog T. The use of botanicals during pregnancy and lactation. *Altern Ther Health Med* 2009;15:54–58.

55. McGuffin M, Hobbs C, Upton R, et al. *American Herbal Products Association's Botanical Safety Handbook.* CRC Press, Boca Raton, FL, 1997.

56. Kauppila A, Kivinen S, Ylikorkala O. A dose response relation between improved lactation and metoclopramide. *Lancet* 1981;1:1175–1157.

57. Milsom SR, Breier BH, Gallaher BW, et al. Growth hormone stimulates galactopoiesis in healthy lactating women. *Acta Endocrinol* 1992;127:337–343.

58. Gunn AJ, Gunn TR, Rabone DL, et al. Growth hormone increases breast milk volumes in mothers of preterm infants. *Pediatrics* 1996;98:279–282.

59. Kaplan W, Sunehag AL, Dao H, et al. Short-term effects of recombinant human growth hormone and feeding on gluconeogenesis in humans. *Metabolism* 2008;57:725–732.

60. Milsom SR, Rabone DL, Gunn AJ, et al. Potential role for growth hormone in human lactation insufficiency. *Horm Res* 1998;50:147–150.

61. Aono T, Aki T, Koike K, et al. Effect of sulpiride on poor puerperal lactation. *Am J Obstet Gynecol* 1982;143:927–932.

62. Ylikorkala O, Kauppila A, Kivinen S, et al. Sulpiride improves inadequate lactation. *BMJ* 1982;285:249–251.

63. Peters R, Schulze-Tollert J, Schuth W. Thyrotophin-releasing hormone—a lactation-promoting agent? *Br J Obstet Gynecol* 1991;98:880–885.

64. Bose CL, D'Ercole AJ, Lester AG, et al. Relactation by mothers of sick and premature infants. *Pediatrics* 1981;67: 565–569.

65. Tyson JE, Perez A, Zanartu J. Human lactational response to oral thyrotropin releasing hormone. *J Clin Endocrinol Metab* 1976;43:760–768.

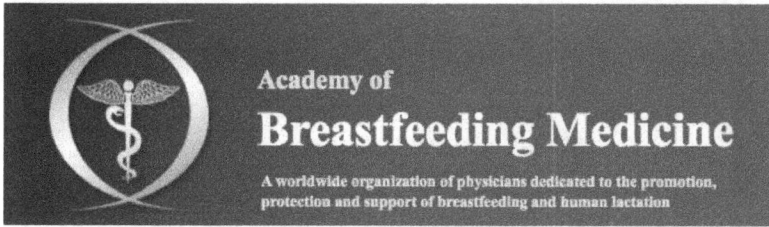

ABM protocols expire 5 years from the date of publication. Evidence-based revisions are made within 5 years or sooner if there are significant changes in the evidence.

Academy of Breastfeeding Medicine Protocol Committee

Maya Bunik, MD, MSPH, FABM

Caroline J. Chantry, MD, FABM

Cynthia R. Howard, MD, M.P.H., FABM

Ruth A. Lawrence, MD, FABM

Kathleen A. Marinelli, MD, FABM, Committee Chairperson

Larry Noble, MD, FABM, Translations Chairperson

Nancy G. Powers, MD, FABM

Julie Scott Taylor, MD, M.Sc., FABM

Contributors

Nancy G. Powers, MD

Anne M. Montgomery, MD

For correspondence
abm@bfmed.org

Appendix: Specific Galactogogues

TABLE 1. POSSIBLY EFFECTIVE FOR SELECTED INDICATIONS

	Domperidone	Fenugreek	Metoclopramide	Silymarin[a]
References	11,44,45,46-52	31,32,53-55	16-20,22-25,56	31,53
Chemical class or properties	Dopamine antagonist	A commonly used spice; active constituents are trigonelline, 4-hydroxyisoleucine, and sotolon.	Dopamine antagonist	Flavolignans (presumed active ingredient)
Level of evidence	I (one study); other studies have inadequate methodology or excessive dropout rates	II-3 (one study in lactating women—abstract only)	III (mixed results in low-quality studies; effect on overall rate of milk secretion is unclear)	II-1 (one study in lactating women)
Suggested dosage	10 mg, orally, 3 times/day in the Level I study; higher doses have not been studied in this context.	"3 capsules," orally (typically 580-610 mg, but not stated in article), 3-4 times/day; strained tea, 1 cup, 3 times/day (¼ tsp of seeds steeped in 8 oz of water for 10 minutes)	10 mg, orally, 3-4 times/day	Micronized silymarin, 420 mg, orally, per day, in study of diPietro et al;[31] anecdotal, strained tea (simmer 1 tsp of crushed seeds in 8 oz of water for 10 minutes), 2-3 cups/day[54]
Length/duration of therapy	Started between 3 and 4 weeks postpartum and given for 14 days in the Level I study. In various other studies the range was considerable. Domperidone was started between 16 to 117 days postpartum and given for 2-14 days.	1 week	7-14 days in various studies	Micronized Silymarin was studied for 63 days.
Herbal considerations	—	Need reliable source of standard preparation without contaminants	—	Need reliable source of standard preparation without contaminants
Effects on lactation	Increased rate of milk secretion for pump-dependent mothers of premature infants less than 31 weeks' gestation in neonatal intensive care unit	Insufficient evidence; likely a significant placebo effect	Possible increased rate of milk secretion; possible responders versus non-responders	Inconclusive
Untoward effects	Maternal: Dry mouth, headache (resolved with decreased dosage), and abdominal cramps. Although not reported in studies of lactation, cardiac arrhythmias are a concern and are occasionally fatal. This may occur with either oral[44] or intravenous	Generally well tolerated. Diarrhea (most common), unusual body odor similar to maple syrup, cross-allergy with Asteraceae/Compositae family (ragweed and related plants), peanuts, and Fabaceae family such as chickpeas, soybeans, and green peas—possible anaphylaxis.	Reversible CNS effects with short-term use, including sedation, anxiety, depression/anxiety/agitation, motor restlessness, dystonic reactions, extrapyramidal symptoms. Rare reports of tardive dyskinesia (usually	Generally well tolerated; occasional mild gastrointestinal side effect; cross-allergy with Asteraceae/Compositae family (ragweed and related plants)—possible anaphylaxis

(continued)

TABLE 1. Continued

	Domperidone	Fenugreek	Metoclopramide	Silymarin[a]
	administration and particularly with high doses, or concurrent use of drugs that inhibit domperidone's metabolism (see Interactions, below). Neonatal: Very low levels in milk and no QTc prolongation in premature infants who had ingested breastmilk of mothers on domperidone.[45]	Theoretically: asthma, bleeding, dizziness, flatulence, hypoglycemia, loss of consciousness, skin rash, wheezing—but no reports in lactating women.	irreversible), causing the FDA to place a "black box warning" on this drug in the United States.	
Interactions	Increased blood levels of domperidone when combined with some substrates metabolized by CYP3A4 enzyme inhibitors, e.g., fluconazole, grapefruit juice, ketoconazole, macrolide antibiotics, and others	Hawthorne, hypoglycemics including insulin, antiplatelet drugs, aspirin, heparin, warfarin, feverfew, primrose oil, many other herbals	Monoamine oxidase inhibitors, tacrolimus, antihistamines, any drugs with CNS effects (including antidepressants)	Caution with CYP2C9 substrates—may increase levels of the drugs. Possible increased clearance of estrogens (decreased blood levels). Possible increased levels of statins. No prescription required
Comments	a. Do not advise exceeding maximum recommended dosage; no increased efficacy but increased untoward effects. b. Generally licensed for use as drug for gastrointestinal dismotility (not in the United States), where for this indication in some regions it is accepted that if no response at the initial dose may increase the dose. Some areas use as drug of choice when prolactin stimulation is felt to be needed. However, there are no studies of the safety or efficacy of this practice in lactating women. c. In the United States, the FDA has issued an advisory *against* the use of domperidone in lactating women.[46]	If patient develops diarrhea, reducing the dose is often helpful.	Some studies suggest tapering off the dose at the end of treatment.	

[a]Silymarin (micronized Silymarin) or *S. marianum* (milk thistle).
CNS, central nervous system; CYP, cytochrome c; FDA, Food and Drug Administration.

TABLE 2. CONTROVERSIAL OR NOT RECOMMENDED, ALTHOUGH POSSIBLY EFFECTIVE

	Human growth hormone	Sulpiride	Thyrotropin-releasing hormone
References	57–60	61,62	19,61,64,65
Chemical class or properties	Protein-based polypeptide hormone: Stimulates multiple growth, anabolic, and anticatabolic effects	Substituted benzamide (antipsychotic, antidepressant); antagonism of presynaptic inhibitory dopamine receptors	A tripeptide hormone that stimulates the release of TSH and prolactin by the anterior pituitary
Level of evidence	Level I[57,58] Level II[59]	II-1 (only two studies)	Level I[63]
Suggested dosage	0.2 IU/kg/day, given intramuscularly or subcutaneously	50 mg, orally, 2 times/day,[59] do not use higher doses because of sedation of mother and baby	1 mg 4 times daily by nasal spray
Length/duration of therapy	7 days, starting anywhere from 8 to 18 weeks postpartum	4-day course starting at 3 days postpartum,[59] no evidence to use for a longer course of treatment	10 days
Effects on lactation	Increased milk secretion in a selected population of normally lactating women with no feeding problems and with healthy thriving infants between 8 and 18 weeks postpartum	Increase in milk secretion in a selected population: Primiparous women with "total yield of milk not exceeding 50 mL for the first 3 postpartum days"	Increased milk secretion in elected population of primiparous women with insufficient milk supply at 5 days postpartum
Untoward effects	None observed in mothers or babies studied to date. Potentially: Joint swelling, joint pain, carpal tunnel syndrome, and an increased risk of diabetes, heart disease	Severe drowsiness; extrapyramidal effects listed in Table 1 for metoclopramide; weight gain	Elevated TSH and hyperthyroidism
Interactions	Other hormones including contraceptives, insulin, cortisol, and others too numerous to list	Levodopa, other drugs with CNS effects	Other hormones including contraceptives, insulin, cortisol, and others too numerous to list
Comments	Insufficient study; not practical—requires injection and is very expensive	Concern about untoward effects	Insufficient study; very expensive; no commercial product available

TSH, thyroid-stimulating hormone.

USLCA

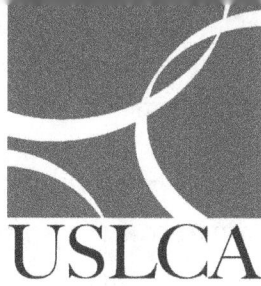

Clinical Decision Making?

When to Consider Using a Nipple Shield

Diane C. Powers, BA, IBCLC, RLC[1]
Vicki Bodley Tapia, BS, IBCLC, RLC[2]

Keywords: Nipple shields, tongue-tie, receding jaw, cephalhematoma, prematurity, sore nipples, flat/inverted nipples, hyperlactation, sexual abuse

Nipple shields have a long and somewhat controversial history. Nearly every published article in recent years reports positive breastfeeding outcomes for mother/baby dyads who used a nipple shield. Their use may be warranted if infants have sucking difficulties, or are having problems latching to flat or inverted nipples.

1   Billings Clinic, dpowers@billingsclinic.org

2   Children's Clinic, victorialee37@gmail.com

In addition, they can be useful for mothers who dread breastfeeding because of nipple pain, are experiencing hyperlactation, or have histories of sexual abuse. It is time to recognize the possible uses for nipple shields that can help create favorable results for breastfeeding couplets.

Although the nipple shield has existed, in one form or another, for centuries, attitudes toward its use as a breastfeeding tool have been mixed. In recent years, some lactation consultants have reported being belittled by colleagues in their work settings for using nipple shields as an intervention in challenging breastfeeding situations. As recently as the Fall of 2010 in the authors' city, WIC contracted with a traveling lactation education group to provide breastfeeding teaching to WIC personnel. The women who attended this educational offering reported to the authors that they were cautioned to never use a nipple shield, being admonished that only inferior lactation consultants resorted to offering nipple shields to breast-feeding mothers.

Descriptions of the device appeared in medical papers in Europe around 1550. Written records show that during that century nipple shields were devised from glass, pewter, tin, horn, or bone (Riordan & Auerbach, 2005). It is difficult to imagine how nipple shields made from these materials were helpful, since they block the suckling stimulus to nerve receptors in the areola, which causes oxytocin release from the pituitary, which provides the neurological underpinning of lactation. Knowing the history of nipple shields allows us to understand that poor suck, flat or inverted nipples, and sore nipples have impacted women's experiences of breastfeeding for hundreds of years.

Nipple shields have evolved through the centuries.

Around 1850, nipple shields began to be made of rubber, and around 1950, latex nipple shields became available. Latex is a stabilized rubber that can be made much thinner than earlier rubber products. Latex nipple shields were probably still too thick for most infants to be able to stimulate the areola sufficiently to send appropriate signals via the breast-brain nerve pathway. Thus, infants using these devices did not always gain suitably.

In 1983, silicone nipple shields appeared on the market. Silicone shields are thinner, extremely pliable, and more malleable than other substances used previously for nipple shields. The introduction of silicone nipple shields provided a tool that could help sustain *at the breast* feeding without causing a decrease in maternal milk supply.

Paula Meier and colleagues published research (Meier, no date; Meier et al., 2006) that showed premature infants with feeding difficulties were able to transfer four times as much milk when a mother used a silicone nipple shield during a feeding, as compared to not using a nipple shield. This was validated with experiments done at two different NICUs in two different states using pre- and post-feed weights of the premature infants. If premature infants are able to sustain sucking and transfer milk better with a nipple shield, then it is reasonable to hypothesize that other infants with suckling difficulties can have a similar result.

Two articles published in the *Journal of Human Lactation* studied nipple-shield use. In the case report, all babies gained the appropriate amount of weight, or better, at 3 weeks, 2 months, and 4 months (Bodley & Powers, 1996). In the 2004 study, 88% of the 200 women interviewed felt the nipple shield helped them breastfeed, and 98% stated they would use the nipple shield again with subsequent children if needed (Powers & Bodley Tapia, 2004). Nipple shields can be used in several different situations.

Situations That May Warrant the Use of Nipple Shield

Infants with Inadequacies in Their Suck Due To Tongue-Tie, a Receding Jaw, Painful Cephalhematoma, or Prematurity

Infants with these issues often transfer an ounce or less, as measured by a pre- and post-feed weight on an electronic scale designed for test weighing. Usually, their weight is already trending downward, with more than a 10% loss from their birth weight. A nipple shield may be used for the next feeding attempt, with pre- and post-feed weights to identify any improvement in milk transfer using the nipple shield. If the infant transfers more milk with the shield, the shield can be used until the infant is able to transfer adequate milk without it. This generally happens as the infant takes in more calories, often improving the sucking coordination and strength. There is no timetable for the infant's readiness.

Painful Nipples Where the Mother Says She Dreads Every Feeding

By covering the damaged nipple, the shield may reduce further injury, thereby speeding healing. Remind the mother that even with the shield, the first minute or two of breastfeeding might still be painful, but after that the pain should subside. When using the nipple shield for abraded nipples, the mother uses the shield until the nipples have healed, with occasional use thereafter, as needed. When nipples have been severely damaged, it is imperative to address the underlying cause of the soreness, most often incorrect latch and/or positioning of the infant, so that when the shield is discontinued, abrasion to the tender nipple skin is not repeated.

For Women Who Have Very Flat Nipples or Inverted Nipples

If women are aware prior to delivery that this anatomical situation might prevent the infant from maintaining a latch, they may have been wearing breast shells for the last four weeks of pregnancy, providing there was no history of pre-term labor. Based on the authors' study of 200 breastfeeding women, breast shells helped to evert nipples approximately 50% of the time prior to the infant's birth (Powers & Bodley Tapia, 2004). Many pregnant women are not aware of the importance of nipple anatomy for ease of breastfeeding until they have difficulty and seek assistance after delivery. This mother may need a nipple shield until the nipples are more easily graspable by the infant, or the infant develops greater sucking strength and coordination to maintain a latch on nipples with less-than-ideal elasticity.

For Women with Hyperlactation

If the mother produces a copious amount of milk, it can cause a newborn infant to choke, sputter, and pull away from the breast, sometimes turning red and struggling to breathe. This phenomenon is alarming to the mother and infant. Depending upon the child's disposition, some infants will even go on a nursing strike when faced with a too-rapid milk flow.

A mother may find using a nipple shield will slow the flow of the milk into a more manageable quantity for the infant, since there are only four holes in the nipple shield, rather than a spray of milk from approximately 7 to 15 nipple pores. The nipple shield is thus used to keep the baby breastfeeding with ease while the mother simultaneously downregulates her milk supply.

Infants may handle high milk flow better if fed in an upright position, straddling the mother's thigh, or prone on a mom lying flat on her back. Milk production can be reduced by breastfeeding on one breast only per feed. If these techniques are insufficient to improve feeding within several days, the mother may increase the amount of hours spent breastfeeding on alternating sides. Some mothers find if they feed the infant on just one breast per feeding, for as many as 12 hours, alternating with the other breast, they will successfully diminish the milk supply within several days.

A mother might also take the original Sudafed containing pseudoephedrine, as directed, for a couple of days to help downregulate her supply. (Note: This is an off-label use of a medication that is non-prescription, but kept behind the counter of pharmacies. It should not be used by women with hypertension, heart disease, or who are taking an MAOI antidepressant, or are allergic to any of the ingredients.) Once the milk supply decreases, the mother would no longer need a nipple shield to manage the milk flow.

For Women with a History of Sexual Abuse

These women may manifest a myriad of breastfeeding outcomes (Bernshaw & Johnson, 1997). Some absolutely can't face breastfeeding, while others share that they are not going to let their perpetrator do further harm by not allowing them to provide the very best nourishment for their infants. Still others find that having the infant on the bare breast is intolerable, even with distraction. But if a nipple shield is used as a barrier between the breast and the infant's mouth, they are able to sustain breastfeeding. For other mothers, this barrier is insufficient and they choose to pump and bottle-feed their milk.

How to Fit a Nipple Shield

According to a widely used nipple-shield manufacturer's instructions:

> The shield should be placed over the breast so that your nipple fits into the nipple chamber of the shield.

It has been our experience that many premature babies with small mouths are able to open their mouths wide enough to attach to the 24 mm nipple shield. We recommend that the nipple shield be fitted to the size of the mother's nipples, not the size of the baby's mouth. Certainly the smaller diameter nipple shields (16 mm or 20 mm) are suitable for women with smaller nipples. If, however, one attempts to only fit the shield to a baby's mouth, and the diameter of that mother's nipples is wider than the teat of the nipple shield, the nipple cannot fully descend into the teat, resulting in less milk transferred. This is not unlike when one pinches a straw and then attempts to suck through it: there is less flow through the crimped straw. The mother's nipples are also at risk for abrasion from the friction caused by rubbing against the interior of the teat that is too small.

Conclusion

There have been 14 articles published regarding nipple shield use since 1990. Thirteen of these articles contained information that supported use of thin silicone nipple shields as an effective clinical intervention in certain situations, also commenting that most women appreciated having this tool in order to keep their infant feeding at the breast (Brigham, 1996; Chertok et al., 2006; Chertok, 2009; Wilson-Clay, 1996).

The thin silicone nipple shield has been available to new mothers for the last quarter century. It is time to recognize the possible uses for nipple shields that can help create positive outcomes for breastfeeding couplets.

References

Bodley, V., & Powers, D. (1996). Long-term nipple shield use—A positive perspective. *Journal of Human Lactation, 12,* 301-304.

Brigham, M. (1996). Mothers' reports of the outcome of nipple shield use. *Journal of Human Lactation, 12,* 291-297.

Chertok, IR. (2009). Reexamination of ultra-thin nipple shield use, infant growth, and maternal satisfaction. *Journal of Clinical Nursing, 18,* 2949-2955.

Chertok, I.R., Schneider, J., & Blackburn, S. (2006). A pilot study of maternal and term infant outcomes associated with ultra-thin nipple shield use. *Journal Obstetrics Gynecology Neonatal Nursing, 35*(2), 265-72.

Meier, P., Brown, L., Hurst, N., et al. (2006). Nipple shields for preterm infants: Effect on milk transfer and duration of breastfeeding. *Journal of Human Lactation, 16,* 106-114.

Meier P. (no date). *Breastfeeding your premature baby using a nipple shield.* Rush-Presbyterian St. Luke's Medical Center, Rush Mothers' Milk Club Special Care Nursery. http://www.medelabreastfeedingus.com/tips-and-solutions/132/breastfeeding-yourpremature-baby-using-a-nipple-shield

Powers, D., & Bodley Tapia, V. (2004). Women's experiences using a nipple shield. *Journal of Human Lactation, 20*(3), 327-334.

Riordan, J., & Auerbach, K. (2005). *Breastfeeding and human lactation, 2nd ed.* Sudbury, MA: Jones & Bartlett Publishers.

Wilson-Clay, B. (1996). Clinical use of silicone nipple shields. *Journal of Human Lactation, 12,* 279-285.

For Further Reading

Clum, D., & Primono, J. (1996). Use of a silicone nipple shield with premature infants. *Journal of Human Lactation, 12,* 287-290.

Drazin, P. (1998). Taking nipple shields out of the closet. *Birth Issues, 7,* 2.

Elliott, C. (1996). Using a silicone nipple shield to assist a baby unable to latch. *Journal of Human Lactation, 12,* 309-313.

Sealy, C. (1996). Rethinking the use of nipple shields. *Journal of Human Lactation, 12,* 299-300.

Woodworth, M., & Frank, E. (1996). Transitioning to the breast at six weeks: Use of a nipple shield. *Journal of Human Lactation, 12,* 305-307.

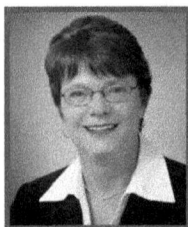

Diane Powers, BA, IBCLC, RLC, is a lactation consultant and former La Leche League leader. For the past 23 years, she has worked with approximately 700 new mother/baby pairs per year, both in-patient and outpatient. She has completed two research projects and had numerous articles published. She lectures nationally and internationally.

Vicki Bodley Tapia, B.S., IBCLC, RLC, is a former La Leche League Leader, and has been in private practice as a lactation consultant since 1987, published numerous articles, and lectures both nationally and internationally. She is the author of *Somebody Stole My Iron: A Family Memoir of Dementia* from Praeclarus Press.

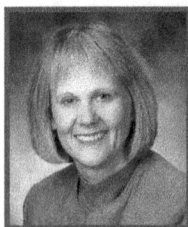

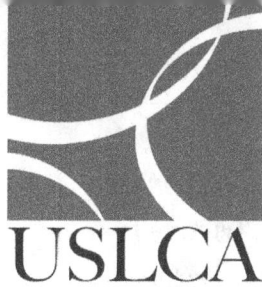

The Effect of Fenugreek on Milk Production and Prolactin Levels in Mothers of Preterm Infants

Carol Reeder, BSN, RN, IBCLC, RLC[1]

Anita LeGrand, BSN, RN[2]

Susan K. O'Connor-Von, PhD, RN[3]

Keywords: Fenugreek, lactation, preterm infant, prolactin

Since 1980, the incidence of preterm birth has increased in the United States. The health importance of human milk is well-known. However, mothers of preterm infants are often concerned that they may not produce enough milk for their infants who

1   St. Luke's Hospital, Cedar Rapids, IA
2   St. Luke's Hospital, Cedar Rapids, IA
3   ocon0025@umn.edu, University of Minnesota, School of Nursing, Minneapolis, MN

are frequently too immature to breastfeed. The herb fenugreek (Trigonella foenum-graecum) is purported to be an effective galactagogue. This double-blind placebo-controlled study sought to determine if fenugreek increased breast milk volume and prolactin (PRL) levels in mothers of preterm infants. The sample included 26 mothers of infants less than 31 weeks gestation. Commencing on the fifth postpartum day, each mother consumed 3 capsules of fenugreek (or placebo), 3 times per day for 21 days. Data analysis revealed no statistical difference between the mothers receiving fenugreek or those receiving placebo in terms of milk volume or PRL. No adverse effects were noted in the mothers or infants.

The incidence of preterm birth has increased by 36% since the 1980s. More than 540,000 premature infants are born each year in the U.S. (National Center for Health Statistics, 2013). Preterm birth is the leading cause of death in newborns, and those who survive often face health challenges (March of Dimes, 2011). The importance of human milk for preterm infants is well known. Breastfed infants have improved enteral feeding tolerance, protection from nosocomial infections, and necrotizing enterocolitis (NEC) when compared with formula-fed infants (Schanler, 2001). According to the American Academy of Pediatrics (AAP; 2005):

Preterm infants receive significant benefits from breast milk, such as a decrease in the incidence and/or severity of infectious diseases, reduced post-neonatal infant mortality rates, decreased rates of sudden infant death syndrome in the first year of life, type 1 and 2 diabetes, lymphoma, leukemia, Hodgkin disease, obesity, hypercholesterolemia and asthma, as well as slightly enhanced performance on cognitive development. (pp. 496–497)

Fenugreek

Herbs and medicinal plants, such as fenugreek (*Trigonella foenum-graecum*), have been used since ancient times (National Institutes of Health, 2012). Hippocrates considered it a soothing herb. Fenugreek is a Greek hayseed originating in the Mediterranean, Southern Europe, and Western Asia (Altuntas, Ozgoz, & Taser, 2005). The aromatic clover-like herb has foliage that grows to 50 cm in height. The pods, containing 5–20 seeds, form as the plant matures. The plant is harvested whole and sundried. The pods are then threshed, and the seeds are used whole or ground. Fenugreek seeds contain 50% fiber (30% soluble fiber and 20% insoluble fiber; Basch, Ulbricht, Kuo, Szapary, & Smith, 2003). One hundred grams of fenugreek contains 26.2 g of protein, 5.8 g of fat, 44.1 g of carbohydrate, and 333 Kcal (Nutritive Value of Indian Spices, 2011). Fenugreek is a natural source of iron, silicon, sodium, and thiamine (Encyclopedia of Spices, 2008).

Fenugreek has been used medicinally as a poultice for skin problems, and as a tea for relief of gastrointestinal upset. Women around the world consume fenugreek seeds to facilitate lactation during the postpartum period

(National Institutes of Health, 2012; National Library of Medicine's LactMed Database, 2012).

Although the exact mechanism for how fenugreek may work is not fully understood, the seed contains hormone precursors that may increase milk production. Its steroidal sapogenins (diosgenin, yamogenin, gitogenin, tigogenin, and neotigogen) and mucilaginous fiber are thought to account for many of the beneficial effects of fenugreek (Drug Information Online, 2013). It is believed that fenugreek stimulates sweat production. Because breasts are modified sweat glands, one hypothesis is that this is how fenugreek increases milk production (Jensen, 2012).

Fenugreek and Breastfeeding

The literature of fenugreek use during lactation contains only a few anecdotal reports of fenugreek use during lactation. A nonblinded, anecdotal study of 1,200 women breastfeeding term infants found that nearly all of those who took fenugreek reported an increase in milk production within 24–72 hours after beginning the herb along with using an electric breast pump (K. Huggins, personal communication, July 1, 2013).

These mothers noted that fenugreek could be discontinued once milk production was stimulated to an appropriate level. No negative side effects in these mothers or infants were reported. Huggins has found fenugreek to be a potent stimulator of breast milk production that appears safe for the mother and baby. However, this study was not reported in the literature. And there have been no studies with mothers of preterm infants, a population that is often concerned about producing enough milk (Hiller-vik-Lindquest, Hofvander, & Sjölin, 1991).

In summary, the benefits of breastfeeding are well established, especially for preterm infants. To date, there are no current published studies examining fenugreek's effect on breast milk volumes or PRL levels in mothers of preterm infants. Therefore, the purpose of this study was to determine if fenugreek increased breast milk volumes and PRL levels in mothers of preterm infants.

Methods

Sample

For this study, a convenience sample of 26 mothers of preterm infants 31 weeks or less gestation was recruited at a Midwestern urban medical center. A multidisciplinary team consisting of a lactation consultant (LC), pediatric registered nurse (RN), pediatrician, neonatologist, obstetrician, neonatal nurse practitioner, pharmacist, laboratory supervisor, and statistician discussed and designed the study. The LC and pediatric RN served as coinvestigators of the study, and completed all recruitment, data collection, and data management. Inclusion criteria consisted of mothers:

a. of infants born 31 weeks or less gestation because these infants would not be breastfeeding,

b. 18 years of age or older,

   c. able to speak and write English,

   d. who began pumping breast milk within 12 hours of delivery,

   e. who had access to a telephone, and

   f. who were able to visit their hospitalized infant daily.

Exclusion criteria included a history of:

   a. infertility,

   b. lack of prenatal breast growth,

   c. breast surgery (excluding breast augmentation),

   d. smoking,

   e. allergy to chickpeas or peanuts,

   f. endocrine problems including diabetes or thyroid disorders, and

   g. taking steroids for any diagnosis other than preterm labor.

Procedure/Data Collection Process

Ethics approval to conduct this study was obtained from the institutional review board at the hospital. All data were stored in a locked file in the LC's office. All personal identifiers were removed and a code number was assigned to every participant.

   The co-investigators reviewed charts daily for mothers who met the inclusion criteria. The first contact was made at the Level II neonatal intensive care unit (NICU) within 4 days post-delivery. Each mother was interviewed to determine final eligibility. At that time, a thorough overview of the study including potential risks to mother and preterm infant, voluntary nature of participation, and the right to withdraw at any time was discussed with each mother. If the mother agreed to participate, the consent form was reviewed, signed, and a copy is left with the mother. Next, the mother was given a demographic questionnaire to complete.

Fenugreek

All mothers were provided with verbal and written information about fenugreek.

Fenugreek (or placebo made of starch) was provided by one consistent, independent pharmacy. A pharmacist randomized whether the fenugreek or placebo was to be administered to the mother using a double-blind procedure, thus the coinvestigators were blind to randomization. Each mother was instructed to take three capsules of 575 mg of fenugreek (or placebo) by mouth three times a day for 21 days, starting after the first PRL level was drawn on the fifth postpartum day.

Breast Pumping

A co-investigator taught the mother the correct usage of the electric breast pump (Lactina®) with a double collection kit, using a comfortable suction setting. The cycling frequency was kept constant at the medium setting. Each mother was instructed to pump 8–10 times a day for 21 days.

Prolactin (PRL) Levels

Mothers were instructed to have three PRL levels drawn at 9:45 a.m. every 5–7 days during the 21-day period. Mothers were instructed to pump before the lab draw. Each serum sample was transported to an independent laboratory for testing. The co-investigators received and recorded the PRL levels according to participant code number.

Logbook

All mothers were instructed to record by hand study information in a logbook over the 21-day period.

The logbook included daily recordings of frequency and time spent (in minutes) pumping, volume of breast milk expressed, time spent in skin-to-skin contact (kangaroo care) with their preterm infant, and any side effects or illnesses the mother experienced.

Perceived Stress/Sleep/Energy/Calmness Scale

The birth of a preterm infant can be highly distressing experience. Psychological distress can be exhibited as perceived stress, inability to sleep, and lack of energy (Hill, Aldag, Chatterton, & Zinaman, 2005b).

To examine psychological distress and its possible effect on milk production, each mother was instructed to record every evening the amount of stress, sleep, energy, and calmness they experienced that day using the Perceived Stress/Sleep/Energy/Calmness Scale. (Permission for use was granted by Pamela D. Hill.) Mothers rated their daily stress, sleep, energy, and calmness on a scale of 0 (*lowest*) to 10 (*highest*).

Infant Data Sheet

An infant data sheet was placed in the medical charts of each preterm infant whose mothers were participating in this study. A NICU nurse practitioner, along with the NICU nursing staff, closely monitored all infants in the study for any untoward symptoms or negative side effects that may have been related to the fenugreek.

On this daily flowsheet, nurses recorded any:

a. change in infant's health,

b. emesis,

c. increase in enteral feeding residuals,

d. abdominal distention,

e. increase in number of apnea/bradycardia spells,

f. loose stools or constipation,

g. change in odor of bodily fluids,

h. rash, or

i. other signs or symptoms.

Data Analysis

Data analysis was performed using *t*-tests and Pearson's correlation on mothers who continued to pump the full 21 days, and that were in compliance with the established study protocol. Analysis of variance was used to compare breast milk volume before and after the use of fenugreek as well as the time of day the breast milk volumes increased. The number of pumpings per day, volume of milk pumped, and PRL levels were compared to the mothers receiving fenugreek versus the mothers receiving placebo. Analysis of the effects of multipara versus primiparous were noted and compared with the amount of milk pumped and PRL levels.

Results

Sample

A convenience sample of 58 mothers met the inclusion criteria and was invited to participate in the study. Although all 58 mothers consented to participate, only 44% ($n = 26$) completed the study. Reasons for not completing the study included missing PRL levels, failure to return the logbook, or transfer of their infant to another healthcare facility.

Maternal and Infant Characteristics

Demographic information for mothers and infants is presented in Table 1. As noted, a higher percentage of mothers taking the fenugreek had prior pregnancies, but not all had prior breastfeeding experience. The average age of mothers in the fenugreek group was younger than those receiving the placebo. The mothers in the experimental group also had higher household incomes (57% earned more than $50,000), and 92% were White.

Table 1. Maternal and Infant Characteristics of the Sample		
Variable	Experimental Group $N = 14$	Placebo Group $N = 12$
Mother:		
Age (years)/(SD)	25.79 (+ 3.98)	27.42 (± 5.79)
Education (years)/(SD)	14.93 (± 1.77)	13.92 (± 1.16)
Income ≥$50,000	8/14 (57%)	6/12 (50%)
Ethnicity/race		
White (non-Hispanic)	13 (92%)	10 (83%)
Black (African American)	0	1
Hispanic	1	1
Prior pregnancy	11/14 (79%)	8/12 (67%)
Prior breastfeeding	2/14 (14%)	3/12 (25%)
Type of delivery		
Vaginal	10	3
Cesarean	4	9
Infant:		
Gender: female	7	4
male	7	8
Age (weeks)/(SD)	27.96 (± 2.30)	28.07 (± 1.85)
Birth weight (grams)/(SD)	1,169 (± 388)	1,222 (± 284)

Difference in Milk Volume

Milk volume totals for Days 5, 10, and 15 are presented in Table 2. The *t*-tests were conducted and the results revealed no statistically significant differences between the average milk volume produced by the fenugreek and placebo groups for any of the three study days.

Difference in PRL Levels

As presented in Table 3, PRL levels were drawn on Days 5, 10, and 15. Two sample *t*-tests revealed no statistically significant difference between the average PRL levels of the mothers receiving fenugreek and the mothers receiving placebo for any of the 3 days. There was no evidence that fenugreek affected the PRL levels for this sample of mothers.

Perceived Stress, Sleep, Energy, and Calmness

None of the four emotion variables had a statistically significant relationship with milk volume. On Day 5, mothers who received fenugreek reported more sleep and energy, as well as less stress in the first 5 days. After Day 5, the results for the mothers receiving fenugreek and those receiving placebo were similar on all four measures. This was unexpected because mothers of preterm infants often appear anxious in the first few days; and as their infant improves, the stress level decreases (Gennaro, York, & Brooten, 1990). A baby suckling at the breast decreases maternal cortisol levels in response to stress (Heinrichs

Table 2. Tests for the Difference in Milk Volume

Day	Group	Total Volume/SD	p Value	Change in Volume/SD	p Value
Day 5	Experimental	345 (± 198)	.645		
	Placebo	391 (± 282)			
Day 10	Experimental	514 (± 351)		169 (± 174)	.811
	Placebo	577 (± 400)		186 (± 205)	
Day 15	Experimental	568 (± 419)		55 (± 102)	.831
	Placebo	622 (± 400)		44 (± 137)	

$p < .05$ (p values of less than .05 would have supported any statistical difference).

Table 3. Tests for the Difference in Prolactin Level

Day	Group	Prolactin/SD	p Value	Change in Volume/SD	p Value
Day 5	Experimental	131.0 (± 128)	.557		
	Placebo	108.9 (± 43.8)			
Day 10	Experimental	97.5 (± 93.4)		−33.2 (± 52.6)	.109
	Placebo	118.5 (±75.1)		9.5 (± 73.4)	
Day 15	Experimental	65.2 (± 67.5)		−32.0 (± 106)	.917
	Placebo	84.9 (± 86.1)		−28.0 (± 116)	

$p < .05$ (p values of less than .05 would have supported any statistical difference).

et al., 2001). Breast pumping, likely, does not provide the same maternal stress reduction as a breastfeeding infant, so milk production may be reduced.

Infant Data

There was no change in the health status and no negative side effects in any of the preterm infants of mothers enrolled in this study.

Discussion

Milk Volume

The purpose of this study was to determine the effect of fenugreek on breast milk volumes and PRL levels in mothers of preterm infants. Although a significant increase in milk volume was not seen in the mothers receiving fenugreek, the exact dose of fenugreek needed by mothers to achieve a desired milk volume remains unclear.

A commonly recommended dose is three capsules (600 mg) three times a day, which usually results in sweat and urine smelling like maple syrup (Hale, 2008). Anecdotally, K. Huggins (personal communication, July 1, 2013) reported that mothers noted an increase in milk production within 24–72 hours.

Prolactin Levels

There was no significant increase in PRL levels in the mothers receiving fenugreek. PRL levels rise during pregnancy, from about 10 ng/ml in the non-pregnant state, to approximately 200–400 ng/ml at term. Baseline levels do not drop back to pre-pregnancy levels in lactating women, but average about 100 ng/ml at 3 months and 50 ng/ml at 6 months (Walker, 2006).

Because the highest concentration of PRL is at night and early morning, when the time between breastfeeding is the longest (Cregan, Mitoulas, & Harmann, 2002), we chose to have the PRL levels drawn after a morning pumping. Zinaman, Hughes, Queenan, Labbok, and Albertson (1992) concluded the PRL levels are higher when mothers used a double-pumping system.

Mothers in this study continued to double-pump for the 21 days they were enrolled. It is well-accepted that an increase in emptying the breast brings about an increase in the rate of milk synthesis over a period of days. Study results showed no difference in milk volume produced by the fenugreek or placebo groups per week.

Frequency of Pumping

Although instructed to pump 8–10 times in 24 hours during the 21 days of study participation, results showed that mothers pumped on average of 5–7 times per 24 hours.

The average milk output for postpartum Days 6 and 7 predicts milk adequacy at 6 weeks postpartum, which reinforces the value of initiating pumping within 6 hours following birth (Hill et al., 2005a). Therefore, it is crucial to teach new mothers that an increase in emptying brings about an increase in the rate of milk synthesis over a period of days. Conversely, decreased emptying brings about a reduction in milk synthesis (Neville, 1999). For this reason, mothers must be instructed about the use of a quality double-breast pump to initiate and maintain adequate milk supply.

New breast pump technologies could impact future studies. Differences in pumping technology, techniques, and instructions can confound milk production studies. Evidence suggests that combining manual expression with electric pumping increases milk production in mothers of preterm infants, along with increasing the caloric content of the milk (Morton et al., 2009; Morton et al., 2012).

Recommendations for Future Research

Future studies of the effect of fenugreek on breast milk volumes and PRL levels in mothers of preterm infants must include a larger, more diverse sample.

A closer evaluation of lactating primiparous versus multiparous mothers is needed to assess if PRL receptors impact overall milk volumes. The onset of pumping before 6 hours is recommended versus 12 hours postdelivery, along with assuring 8–12 pumpings per day. Further evaluation of the effect of prenatal betamethasone on lactation is also needed.

A diet history evaluating caloric intake before and during the study period might shed some light on why, in some regions of the world, fenugreek is reported to be effective in increasing milk volumes. Lastly, a closer examination of mothers' perceived stress, sleep, energy, and calmness is needed along with the involvement of the family, the healthcare team, and the community to nurture these mothers to ensure successful initiation and continuation of lactation.

Conclusion

The importance of human milk for preterm infants is well recognized. The purpose of this study was to examine the use of fenugreek with breastfeeding mothers of preterm infants, and its effect on milk volume and PRL levels.

Fenugreek is one of the most common herbs mothers use in an effort to increase milk volume. However, there is a paucity of research determining its efficacy and safety.

Although there was not a significant difference in breast milk volumes and PRL levels in mothers who received fenugreek versus those who received a placebo, no change in health status or negative side effects were observed in either the mothers or preterm infants.

References

Altuntas, E., Ozgoz, E., & Taser, F. (2005). Some physical properties of fenugreek seeds. *Journal of Food Engineering, 71*, 37–43.

American Academy of Pediatrics. (2005). Breastfeeding and the use of human milk. *Pediatrics, 115*, 496–506.

Basch, E., Ulbricht, C., Kuo, G., Szapary, P., & Smith, M. (2003). Therapeutic applications of fenugreek. *Alternative Medicine Review, 8*, 20–27.

Cregan, M., Mitoulas, L., & Harmann, P. (2002). Milk prolactin, feed volume and duration between feeds in women breastfeeding their full-term infants over a 24-hour period. *Experimental Physiology, 87,* 207–214.

Drug Information Online. (2013). Retrieved from http://www.drugs.com

Encyclopedia of Spices. (2008). Retrieved from http://theepicentre.com/spice/fenugreek/

Gennaro, S., York, R., & Brooten, D. (1990). Anxiety and depression in mothers of LBW and VLBW infants: Birth through 5 months. *Issues in Comprehensive Pediatric Nursing, 13,* 97–109.

Hale, T. (2008). *Medication and mothers' milk.* Amarillo, TX: Hale Publishing.

Heinrichs, M., Meinlschmidt, G., Neumann, I., Wagner, S., Kirschbaum, C., Ehlert, U., & Hellhammer, D. H. (2001). Effects of suckling on hypothalamic-pituitary-adrenal axis responses to psychosocial stress in postpartum lactating women. *Journal of Clinical Endocrinology and Metabolism, 86,* 4798–4804.

Hill, P. D., Aldag, J. C., Chatterton, R. T., & Zinaman, M. (2005a). Comparison of milk output between mothers of preterm and term infants: The first 6 weeks after birth. *Journal of Human Lactation, 21,* 22–30.

Hill, P. D., Aldag, J. C., Chatterton, R. T., & Zinaman, M. (2005b). Psychological distress and milk volume in lactating mothers. *Western Journal of Nursing Research, 27,* 676–693.

Hillervik-Lindquest, C., Hofvander, Y., & Sjölin, S. (1991). Studies on perceived breast milk insufficiency. III. Consequences for breast milk consumption and growth. *ACTA Paediatrica Scandnavica, 80,* 297–303.

Jensen, R. (2012). *Fenugreek: Overlooked but not forgotten.* Retrieved from http://www.breastfeedingonline.com/fenugreekoverlooked.shtml#sthash.5L6MvrK7.dpbs

March of Dimes. (2011). *What's new: Preterm birth.* Retrieved from: http://www.marchofdimes.com

Morton, J., Hall, J., Wong, R., Thairu, L., Benitz, W., & Rhine, W. (2009). Combining hand techniques with electric pumping increases milk production in mothers of preterm infants. *Journal of Perinatology, 29,* 757–764.

Morton, J., Wong, R., Hall, J., Pang, W., Lai, C., Lui, J., . . . Rhine, W. (2012). Combining hand techniques with electric pumping increases the caloric content of milk in mothers of preterm infants. *Journal of Perinatology, 32,* 791–796.

National Center for Health Statistics. (2013). *Preterm birth rates.* Retrieved from http://www.marchofdimes.com/peristats

National Institutes of Health: National Center for Complementary and Alternative Medicine. (2012). *Herbs at a glance: Fenugreek.* Retrieved from http://nccam.nih.gov/health/fenugreek

National Library of Medicine's LactMed Database. (2012). *Fenugreek use while breastfeeding.* Retrieved from http://toxnet.nlm.nih.gov/cgibin/sis/search/f?./temp/~b9ojPO:1

Neville, M. C. (1999). Physiology of lactation. *Clinics in Perinatology, 26,* 251–279.

Nutritive Value of Indian Spices. (2011). Retrieved from http://www.indianspices.com/html/s062mvl1.htm#Fenugreek

Schanler, R. (2001). The use of human milk for premature infants. *Pediatric Clinics of North America, 48,* 207–219.

Walker, M. (2006). *Breastfeeding management for the clinician using the evidence.* Boston, MA: Jones and Bartlett.

Zinaman, M., Hughes, V., Queenan, J. T., Labbok, M. H., & Albertson, B. (1992). Acute prolactin responses and milk yield to infant suckling and artificial methods of expression in lactating women. *Pediatrics, 89,* 437–440.

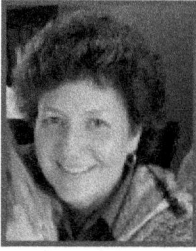

Carol Reeder, BSN, RN, IBCLC, RLC, has worked as a Mother-Baby nurse and lactation consultant at St. Luke's Hospital, Cedar Rapids, Iowa for the past 30 years. She has been an active member of the Iowa Breast-feeding Coalition since 1990, and is presently serving a 2-year term as Coalition Co-Chair.

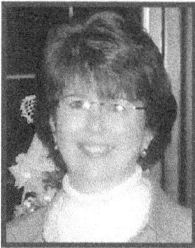

Anita LeGrand, BSN, RN, has worked as a staff nurse in the emergency room in Harlan, Kentucky, and a staff nurse, clinician, and assistant manager in the Pediatric Intensive Care Unit at St. Luke's Hospital in Cedar Rapids, Iowa. Currently she is working in quality management at St. Luke's Hospital.

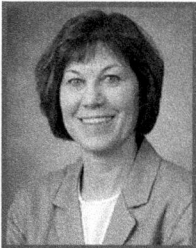

Susan O'Conner-Von, PhD, RN, is Associate Professor of Nursing, University of Minnesota. Her research interests include pediatric pain, palliative care, preparation for surgery, web-based educational programs for adolescents, and spirituality care.

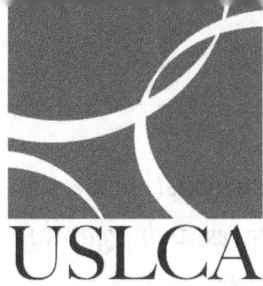

Placenta Medicine as a Galactogogue:
Tradition or Trend?

Melissa Cole, IBCLC, RLC[1]

Keywords: Placenta medicine, galactogogue, placentophagy, human placenta, milk supply

For some mothers, insufficient milk supply impacts their ability to fully breastfeed their infants. Many of these mothers seek holistic options to increase their milk supply. Placenta medicine, or postpartum placenta consumption as a purported galactogogue, appears to be a practice on the rise in the United States. There is some limited historical research, and more recently some phenomenological data, about the practice of placenta as a galactogogue. However, little is truly known about the benefits and risks of placentophagy, in general, or specifically, as a galactogogue.

---

1   melissa@lunalactation.com

This article reviews existing literature and proposes a further call for research regarding the safety and efficacy of placenta consumption.

Placenta medicine usage, or placentophagy, is on the rise. The practice seems to be gaining momentum around the U.S. and abroad. Placentophagy is defined as the consumption of placenta and/or related tissues and membranes. Many mothers consume their placentas, often in capsulated form, for their purported health benefits, including improving mood and boosting milk production.

Many pro–placenta medicine websites cite the same, and a few studies find benefits of placentophagy. Unfortunately, many of the studies cited are nearly 100 years old, and the methodology used in them would not hold up to today's scientific standards. Moreover, there is a lack of updated information regarding placenta consumption among humans, and even less literature on the topic of placenta as a galactogogue.

Because placenta consumption is on the rise, this article has five main goals:

a. to explore whether placentophagy is tradition or trend by reviewing past/present practices,

b. to review the available literature and research on placenta consumption,

c. to explore the ethical aspects of placenta as a galactogogue,

d. to acknowledge ethical considerations around placenta preparation, and

e. to propose a call for research regarding this topic.

Placentophagy in Portland and Beyond

Currently, there are no national U.S. statistics published comparing placentophagy practices by state. A review of approximately 1,000 client intake forms from the past 5 years of my practice showed that up to 50% of my homebirth clients, and up to 10% of the birth center/hospital families, ingested their placenta after delivery.

There are approximately 20,000 live births per year in the Metro Portland area (Oregon Health Authority, 2011), and a 1.96% homebirth rate in Oregon (Centers for Disease Control and Prevention, 2012). This implies that roughly 2,000 mothers per year consume their placenta in Portland alone. One recent study looking at placentophagy primarily in the U.S. and Canada found that homebirth mothers were 25% more likely to engage in placentophagy than mothers delivering in hospitals (Selander, Cantor, Young, & Benyshek, 2013, p. 100).

Most babies in the U.S. are born in the hospital. Nevertheless, there does seem to be a trend regarding increased placenta medicine usage among mothers in many communities worldwide.

Modes of Preparation for Consumption

There are several modes of human placenta preparation for consumption. Encapsulation is the most popular method, with 80% of study participants choosing some form of it (Selander et al., 2013, p. 103). For encapsulation, raw or cooked placenta is dehydrated and then grounded into a powder and put into capsules. Placenta tincture, cooked placenta, raw placenta, and other methods are also used to a lesser degree. With more mothers choosing to consume their placenta, there has been an explosion in the number of professionals including doulas, childbirth educators, and midwives who are providing placenta medicine-making services.

> Although placentophagy is absent in the cross-cultural ethnographic record ... demand for placenta-preparation services and an increase in the numbers of people becoming trained in providing the services may indicate an increasing popularity of, and interest in, the practice. (Selander et al., 2013, p. 94)

This in itself could be a concern because of the lack of oversight on training and preparation of placenta as food.

Reasons Why Mothers Consume Their Placenta

Mothers choose to participate in placentophagy for a variety of reasons. The most commonly identified reasons for placentophagy include maternal desire for improved mood and/or general health benefits; the recommendation from someone, such as a midwife; and the desire to recover from birth, optimize lactation, and replace lost nutrients and minerals (Selander et al., 2013, pp. 101–102).

In a phenomenological study of 189 women who had consumed their placenta (most from the U.S. and Canada, all older than the age 18 years), Selander et al. (2013) found that 92% of participants were positive about their placento-phagy experience and 98% would engage in placentophagy again, even if they had a negative experience. In the Selander et al. study, the women were asked questions about demographic info, why they chose placentophagy, type of placenta preparation they used, and any perception of positive or negative effects.

In an informal survey of my clients, I found that most who engaged in placentophagy felt that it helped their mood/health to some extent, or felt that *it wouldn't hurt, so why not?* There were some mothers who said that they had negative effects. One mother felt like it increased her anxiety.

Despite the fact that placenta consumption does not seem to be the norm for humans, mothers who participate in placentophagy, overwhelmingly, seem to find it beneficial.

Placenta Consumption in Other Mammals

Nonhuman mammals are more likely to consume their placentas. Kristal is one prominent researcher, with articles spanning from 1973 to 2012. For example, Kristal, DiPirro, and Thompson (2012) observed that most nonhuman, peripartum female mammals ingest all or a portion of the afterbirth (the amniotic fluid, the placenta, and/or associated membranes).

Researchers have many hypotheses for why mammals consume their placentas: keeping the nest area clean, reducing odors that may attract predators, replenishing nutrients, acquiring hormones, and responding to general and/or specific hunger (Kristal et al., 2012, p. 179). However, although researchers found some truth in these apparent reasons, they were not able to provide evidence to support these working hypotheses. Therefore, these researchers have speculated that there must be other reasons for placentophagia being the biological norm for most mammals (Noonan & Kristal, 1979).

One important finding regarding placentophagia was the discovery that when rats ingested amniotic fluid and their placentas, it helped them initiate maternal caretaking behavior (Kristal, 2009). Another important finding was that when rats ingested amniotic fluid and their placentas, it enhanced morphine-mediated pain relief, labeled placental opioid-enhancing factor (POEF; Kristal, Abbott, & Thompson, 1988).

This research showed that by ingesting a small amount of amniotic fluid, the mother could receive opioid-enhancing benefits *before* the first fetus was born, and that pain relief could be continued after delivery with ingestion of the placenta (Kristal, Thompson, & Abbott, 1986). Researchers went on to find that POEF did not seem to be species- or gender-specific; POEF seem to provide an analgesic effect to any mammal that consumes another mammal's amniotic fluid and placental tissue orally (Abbott et al., 1991; Kristal et al., 1986; Thompson, Abbott, Doerr, Ferguson, & Kristal, 1991).

Researchers combined these two significant placento-phagia benefits into the idea that:

> The effect of POEF on the parturitional pain threshold seems to be based on an elegantly orches-trated system of behavioral and biochemical events, exquisitely timed, that serves to counter the pain of delivery, partially, without increasing [other chemicals/hormones] that might compromise the mother's health ... or her ability to care for the young. (Kristal et al., 2012, pp. 185–186)

So, it appears that placentophagia among mammals is about more than just replacing nutrients or staving off predators. There seems to be a complex, multifaceted biological imperative for the practice. One anthropological question Kristal and colleagues (2012) have raised is,

> Why don't humans engage in placentophagia as a biological imperative? Is it possible that there is more adaptive advantage in not doing so? (p. 177)

Kristal and colleagues (2012) demonstrated that animals needed to consume raw amniotic fluid and raw placenta to optimize the pain relief and maternal–infant bonding effects. Their studies showed that the beneficial properties in the afterbirth materials were inactivated if left at room temperature for more than 24 hours or heated to greater than 35 °C (Kristal et al., 2012, p. 189). They note that "more afterbirth is not necessarily better ... Larger amounts ingested at one time are not effective or are possibly inhibitory" (Kristal et al., 1988; Kristal, Thompson, & Grishkat, 1985). Given the fact that the most popular human form of placenta consumption (cooked or raw and then dehydrated/ encapsulated and taken for extended periods of time after delivery) is nothing like the raw amniotic fluid/ placenta dose that other mammals consume after birth. Can humans expect any of the same benefits?

Placenta Medicine: Tradition or Trend?

What is the modern and historical cultural norm for consuming one's placenta after birth? One recent study shows that 66% of male and female participants were aware of placentophagy, but only 3.3% had actually consumed placenta (Cremers & Low, 2014).

Even though awareness about the practice of placenta consumption is increasing, historically, humans have only consumed placenta in very rare cases. Researchers have found that the practice has only been increasing in the last 30 years among a very small minority of individuals (Menges, 2007). Although more than 4,000 terrestrial mammal species do ingest their placenta and/or amniotic fluid, researchers hypothesize that the practice of human placentophagia does not seem to be physiologically or phylogenetically based (Menges, 2007; Young & Benyshek, 2010).

In a comprehensive cross-cultural study, Young and Benyshek (2010) examined the beliefs and traditions surrounding the placenta. Out of 179 societies around the globe, placenta consumption was very rare, with only a few isolated cases being noted. Some of the literature did reference the practice of placenta consumption as being advocated by some midwives in Mexico and the U.S. beginning around the 1970s.

A few societies (primarily Vietnamese and Chinese) have traditional human placenta medicines. In traditional chinese medicine (TCM), human placenta is known to:

> Tonify liver and kidneys ... treats deficiency of yin and yang ... nourishes the blood: ... for insufficient lactation due to exhaustion of qi and blood ... Use caution with long term ... only the placentas of women without disease should be used (Bensky, Clavey, & Stöger, 2004, pp. 806–808)

There are many variations of placenta preparation in TCM, often related to the province or location. Toxicity issues concerning placenta medicine have been noted in regards to pharmacological pain management for patients in general. But not necessarily for new mothers.

Placenta as a Galactogogue: What the Literature Shows

International Board Certified Lactation Consultants need to understand how placenta consumption may impact lactation. Proponents of placentophagia claims that placenta consumption can increase milk supply. There is very little evidence to support this claim. McNeile and Hammett were researchers that studied placenta consumption and lactation almost 100 years ago. McNeile, based in a Los Angeles hospital, gave desiccated placenta to eight patients and used another eight patients as the control group and then examined their breast milk and infants' weights. He reported that:

> ... there was apparently some change in the chemical composition of the milk ... an increase in lactose ... a slight increase in protein ... a slight decrease in the percentage of fat. There was no deficiency in the amount of milk in any of the cases receiving desiccated placenta, but the reverse was true in cases which did not receive this agent. There was apparently a slight decrease in the initial loss of weight in the infants of mothers receiving the desiccated placenta, over those whose mothers did not receive it, and at the end of eleven days the babies whose mothers received the agent were about four ounces heavier than those who did not. (McNeile, 1918, pp. 377–383)

Hammett took these ideas a step further and conducted a series of experiments, primarily at Boston Lying-In Hospital (now Brigham and Women's Hospital). For one of his main studies, Hammett collected data on normal growth curves for 537 exclusively breastfed infants whose mothers had not consumed placenta. He collected data on the weights of 177 infants whose mothers were given 10 g of desiccated placenta in capsules three times per day for 2 weeks. He then compared the weights of those 177 babies against the collective growth curve of the original 587 babies whose mothers had not received placenta. He examined the effects of ingested desiccated placenta on infant growth.

Hammett found, based on bedside observation, that changes in breast milk volume or breast tissue growth postplacenta ingestion were not significant. However, he found that there must be some stimulus in the placenta that gets passed through the milk and impacts infant growth (Hammett, 1918, 1919). Hammett described his findings:

> The effect of the ingestion of the placenta by mothers on the growth of the breast-feeding infants is at once apparent ... the rate of growth of the breast-fed infants is enhanced by the maternal ingestion of desiccated placenta, for not only is the recovery to or over the initial weight generally more rapid, but the weight is almost uniformly greater ... A large series of comparative measurements of the mammae of women taking and not taking the desiccated placenta, combined with a study of the time of onset of full milk production, failed to show either hypertrophy of the gland or an increased milk production on the part of those women ingesting the placenta ... we conclude that there must be contained in the desiccated placenta some substance ... capable of passing through the maternal organism ... passed on to the infant in the

milk, acting as stimuli to growth ... these substances in utero may play an important part in the growth of the embryo and fetus. (Hammett, 1918, pp. 570–573)

A 1954 study of 27 mothers (all selected because of suspected low-supply concerns; no control group was used) found that freeze-dried placenta had a positive impact on maternal milk supply among selected study participants (Soykova-Pachnerova, Brutar, Golova, & Zvolska, 1954).

We wanted to help mothers ... our aim was to make good nurses of our mothers ... we can report on 210 women who ate placenta: 71 with very good results, 110 with good, and 29 with negative results ... In evaluating these results we make allowance for the physiological increase in milk during the first days after delivery. It should be borne in mind that the women who received this treatment were those in whom some trouble in nursing was anticipated: women with flat or unglandular breasts or mutliparae who after previous deliveries had nursed badly or not at all ... the effective substance in placenta is not protein. Nor does lyofilised placenta act as a biogenic stimulator ... the question of hormonal influence remains open. So far it could be shown that progesterone is probably not active in increasing lactation ... this method of treating hypogalactia seems worth noting since the placenta preparation is easily obtained, has not so far been utilized and in our experience is successful in the majority of women. (Soykova-Pachnerova et al., 1954, pp. 618–626)

Among animal studies, "There has been documentation of both beneficial and detrimental effects of eating placenta in the lactational period" (Kristal, 1980, p. 16). Some rat studies have shown that placentophagy does in fact impact prolactin and progesterone levels:

> In rats that were allowed to eat the placentae after parturition concentrations of serum prolactin were elevated on Day 1, but concentrations of serum progesterone were depressed on Days 6 and 8 postpartum when compared to those of rats prevented from eating the placentae. In rats treated with PMSG to induce superovulation serum prolactin and progesterone values were significantly ($p < 0.05$) elevated on Days 3 and 5 respectively, after being fed 2 g rat placenta/day for 2 days. However, feeding each rat 4 g placenta/day significantly ($p < 0.02$) lowered serum progesterone on Day 5. Oestrogen injections or bovine or human placenta in the diet had no effect. The organic phase of a petroleum ether extract of rat placenta (2 g-equivalents/day) lowered peripheral concentrations of progesterone on Day 5, but other extracts were ineffective. We conclude that the rat placenta contains orally-active substance(s) which modify blood levels of pituitary and ovarian hormones. (Blank & Friesen, 1980, p. 273)

Even though placentophagy may impact hormones of lactation, very few humans consume raw placenta immediately after delivery (Selander et al., 2013, p. 103). Some hormones and nutrients have been studied in unprepared term placenta, and "While the exact concentration of many of these hormones and nutrients in the placenta is unknown .... It is unclear, however, if the biological components in the placenta remain active after the organ has been prepared for consumption" (Selander et al., 2013, p. 95). Given the variety of, and lack of research on, how preparation methods alter the placenta hormonal/nutrient makeup, it is nearly impossible to extrapolate findings from animal-based research to human placentophagy.

The aforementioned studies are what pro–placenta medicine proponents usually cite. By today's standards, these older studies have methodological flaws, poor control measures, and small samples sizes. The Selander et al. (2013) study is a phenomenological research study with self-selected participants. It does not account for the placebo effect. These studies do add to the literature, but if placenta as a galactogogue is to be taken seriously, it needs more rigorous research, such as double-blind, randomized trials, done in the future. Like Kristal et al. (2012) points out, "by today's scientific standards, we cannot draw meaningful conclusions from [those studies], even if there is a real effect" (Kristal et al., 2012, p. 188). Given the benefits of optimal lactation, and the few pharmacological galactogogues available to mothers coping with insufficient milk supply, exploring placenta medicine is one possible option.

Ethical Concerns Regarding Placenta Preparation and Consumption

Mothers' reports of positive placentophagy experiences cannot be ignored. Even in traditions where placenta medicine is used, there are contraindications and risks associated with the practice that should be examined. Without further research, we cannot be certain what hormones and chemical components remain bioactive after placenta preparation and which mothers may be helped or harmed by them. With more people becoming certified in placenta medicine preparation, what are the legal or ethical considerations?

Can a mother even have legal access to her placenta? Mothers in various states have had to fight for their legal right to keep their placenta following a hospital birth (*Judge orders hospital*, 2007; Lauer, 2006). In such cases, all of the judges ruled to allow the mothers to take home their placenta despite the hospital pleading that it was a biohazard. In these cases, the ethical tenet of autonomy was upheld; the individual's right to be free from deceit, duress, constraint, or coercion (Edge & Groves, 2005, p. 60) was respected. But beyond the concept of simply having access to one's placenta, the idea behind ethical placenta preparation and promotion must be explored.

Veracity and nonmaleficence are basic principles of healthcare ethics. When it comes to veracity, placenta preparation professionals must be honest with themselves and their clients. There may be ample anecdotal evidence about the benefits of placenta consumption, but there is little empirical evidence. Nonmaleficence is often associated with the ancient adage, *primum non nocere* ("above all [or first], do no harm") (Noel-Weiss & Walters, 2006, p. 208). When it comes to doing no harm regarding professional placenta preparation, the preparer must consider the very real possibility of contamination when handling bodily fluids/organs and the client ingesting the preparation.

Upon review, several placenta preparer websites claim to adhere to federal safety guidelines, as well as have training in blood-borne pathogens, and even state-issued food handler cards. It does seem that businesses involved with placenta preparation are trying to be conscientious with their preparations. However, consumers must keep in mind that certification is not required or accredited by any official organization, and there are no regulations or oversight when it comes to placenta medicine at this time. Professionals, and the mothers they serve, should fully understand the risks versus benefits of placenta preparation and consumption to make an informed choice.

Conclusion and Call for Research

With the exception of some traditional, medicinal preparations, human placenta consumption postpartum seems to be a relatively new practice that is currently limited to a small subset of mothers. Biologically active components in various human placenta medicine preparations have not been researched thoroughly.

Even though placentophagia proponents claim that consuming placenta has many health benefits, these claims often come from either outdated research or animal-based research that cannot readily be extrapolated to the modern styles of human placenta consumption. Despite the fact that there is little available evidence for the practice of placentophagia, phenomenological research has shown that most who do consume their placenta find it to be beneficial, and 98% of participants would do it again (Selander et al., 2013). Knowing that many mothers have found benefits from consuming their placenta, we must remember that *absence of proof is not proof of absence* (William Cowper as cited in Kristal et al., 2012, p. 187).

The claims of placentophagia need to be tested more extensively. The existing studies do not account for the placebo effect (i.e., mothers find that it works because they believe that it will). Is it belief alone that accounted for the findings? Does encapsulated placenta have an effect above and beyond the placebo effect? And does it have a negative impact on lactogenesis and/or milk production? Could it have a role in medicinal pain relief in the future? What substances are still bioactive in prepared forms of placenta medicine? There may be additional benefits of placenta consumption and optimal modes of preparation for researchers to discover, but these claims need to be evaluated via rigorous research.

Given the reality that there is little research when it comes to human placenta preparation and consumption, the ethical and legal issues around this topic must be explored further as well. Animal research has certainly shown that there are very real benefits for nonhuman mammalian placentophagy, especially when it comes to pain relief during/after labor and optimizing maternal–infant bonding (Apari & Rozsa, 2006; Kristal, 1980; Kristal et al., 2012).

In addition, limited human research has shown some benefits, such as improved infant weight gain, increased supply in some cases, and overall maternal satisfaction with the practice. The possibilities for potential human applications regarding placenta ingestion certainly warrant a call for research.

Although placenta medicine is still viewed as an obscure, fringe practice by many, some mothers are embracing it. As demand for this practice increases, researchers and healthcare professionals alike will have to invest more time and resources into studying human placentophagy so that we can better understand the clinical applications and risks versus benefits of this practice.

References

Abbott, P., Thompson, A. C., Ferguson, E. J., Doerr, J. C., Tarapacki, J. A., Kostyniak, P. J., . . . Kristal, M. B. (1991). Placental opioid-enhancing factor (POEF): Generalizability of effects. *Physiology & Behavior, 50* (5), 933–940.

Apari, P., & Rozsa, L. (2006). Deal in the womb: Fetal opiates, parent/offspring conflict, and the future of midwifery. *Medical Hypotheses, 67* (5), 1189–1194. http://dx.doi.org/10.1016/j.mehy.2006.03.053

Bensky, D., Clavey, S., & Stöger, E. (2004). *Chinese herbal medicine: Materia medica* (3rd ed.). Seattle, WA: Eastland Press.

Blank, M. S., & Friesen, H. G. (1980). Effects of placentophagy on serum prolactin and progesterone concentrations in rats after parturition or superovulation. *Journal of Reproduction and Fertility, 60* (2), 273–278.

Centers for Disease Control and Prevention. (2012). *Homebirth in the United States.* Retrieved from http://www.cdc.gov/nchs/data/databriefs/db84.pdf

Cremers, G. E., & Low, K. G. (2014). Attitudes toward placentophagy: A brief report. *Health Care for Women International, 35* (2), 113–119. http://dx.doi.org/10.1080/07399332.2013.798325

Edge, R. S., & Groves, J. R. (2005). *Ethics of health care : A guide for clinical practice* (3rd ed.). Clifton Park, NY: Thomson Delmar Learning.

Hammett, F. S. (1918). The effect of the maternal ingestion of desiccated placenta upon the rate of growth of the breast-fed infant. *Journal of Biological Chemistry, 36*, 569–573.

Hammett, F. S. (1919). Internal secretion of the placenta. *Endocrinology, 3*, 307.

Kristal, M. B. (1980). Placentophagia: A biobehavioral enigma (or *De gustibus non disputandum est*). *Neuroscience & Biobehavioral Reviews, 4* (2), 141–150.

Kristal, M. B. (2009). The biopsychology of maternal behavior in nonhuman mammals. *ILAR Journal, 50* (1), 51–63.

Kristal, M. B., Abbott, P., & Thompson, A. C. (1988). Dosedependent enhancement of morphine-induced analgesia by ingestion of amniotic fluid and placenta. *Pharmacology, Biochemistry, and Behavior, 31* (2), 351–356.

Kristal, M. B., DiPirro, J. M., & Thompson, A. C. (2012). Placentophagia in humans and nonhuman mammals: Causes and consequences. *Ecology of Food and Nutrition, 51* (3), 177–197. http://dx.doi.org/10.1080/03670244.2012.661325

Kristal, M. B., Thompson, A. C., & Abbott, P. (1986). Ingestion of amniotic fluid enhances opiate analgesia in rats. *Physiology & Behavior, 38* (6), 809–815.

Kristal, M. B., Thompson, A. C., & Grishkat, H. L. (1985). Placenta ingestion enhances opiate analgesia in rats. *Physiology & Behavior, 35* (4), 481–486.

Judge orders hospital to give mom placenta. (2007, July 18). *Las Vegas Review Journal*. Retrieved from http://www.reviewjournal. com/news/judge-orders-hospital-give-mom-placenta

Lauer, N. (2006, July 28). *Hawaiian law now permits parents to keep placentas.* Retrieved from http://womensenews.org/story/ parenting/060728/hawaiian-law-now-permits-parents-keep-placentas

McNeile, L. G. (1918). Effect of ingestion of desiccated placenta during first 11 days of lactation, preliminary report. *American Journal of Obstetrics and Diseases of Women and Children, 77*, 377–383.

Menges, M. (2007). Evolutional and biological aspects of placentophagia. *Anthropologischer Anzeiger, 65*(1), 97–108.

Noel-Weiss, J., & Walters, G. J. (2006). Ethics and lactation consultants: Developing knowledge, skills, and tools. *Journal of Human Lactation, 22*(2), 203–212; quiz 213–217. http://dx.doi. org/10.1177/0890334406286955

Noonan, M., & Kristal, M. B. (1979). Effects of medial preoptic lesions on placentophagia and on the onset of maternal behavior in the rat. *Physiology & Behavior, 22*(6), 1197–1202.

Oregon Health Authority. (2011). *Births by county and zip code.* Retrieved from http://public.health.oregon.gov/ BirthDeathCertificates/VitalStatistics/birth/Pages/zipcnty.aspx

Selander, J., Cantor, A., Young, S. M., & Benyshek, D. C. (2013). Human maternal placentophagy: A survey of self-reported motivations and experiences associated with placenta consumption. *Ecology of Food and Nutrition, 52*(2), 93–115. http://dx.doi.org/10.1080/03670244.2012.719356

Soykova-Pachnerova, E., Brutar, V., Golova, B., & Zvolska, E. (1954). Placenta as a lactagogon. *Gynaecologia, 138*(6), 617–627.

Thompson, A. C., Abbott, P., Doerr, J. C., Ferguson, E. J., & Kristal, M. B. (1991). Amniotic fluid ingestion before vaginal/ cervical stimulation produces a dose-dependent enhancement of analgesia and blocks pseudopregnancy. *Physiology & Behavior, 50*(1), 11–15.

Young, S. M., & Benyshek, D. C. (2010). In search of human placentophagy: A cross-cultural survey of human placenta consumption, disposal practices, and cultural beliefs. *Ecology of Food and Nutrition, 49*(6), 467–484. http://dx.doi.org/10.1080/03670 244.2010.524106

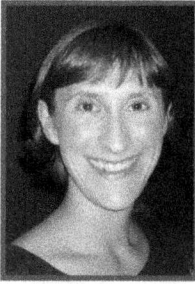

Melissa Cole, IBCLC, RLC, is a board-certified lactation consultant, neonatal oral-motor assessment professional, and wellness clinician in private practice.

Melissa is passionate about providing comprehensive, holistic lactation support. She is dedicated to improving the level of clinical lactation skills for healthcare providers.

She is an adjunct professor at Birthingway College of Midwifery in Portland, Oregon, where she teaches advanced clinical lactation skills. She is active with several lactation and healthcare professional associations including the International Affiliation of Tongue-Tie Professionals.

Melissa lectures, publishes, and conducts research on lactation, herbal medicine, and health-related topics. She is currently co-investigator on an IRB-approved study regarding frenotomy outcomes. Melissa enjoys living and working in the beautiful Pacific Northwest.

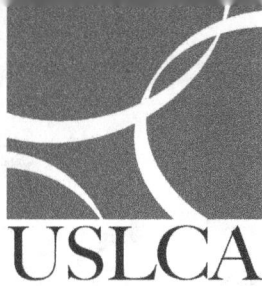

Clinical Tips

Caring for Breast Pump Parts, Cleaning Breast Pump Parts

Kathleen Chiu, IBCLC, RLC[1]

Keywords: Breastfeeding, pumping, pump parts

Many mothers use breast pumps to build or maintain their milk supplies, or to provide their milk for their babies. Breast pumps do require regular care to ensure that they last. This article provides some practical tips for mothers on caring for their breast pumps.

Unless the kit is sterile, a member of the baby's household should clean kit parts before the first use. (*Home germs are best germs.*) The pieces that should normally be washed include the milk storage containers (bottles), the flanges or breast shields, and the valves/membranes.

Pump tubing only requires washing if it gets wet inside. Filters should not be washed either. They are meant

---

1   amcbe@comcast.net

to shut-down if wet to stop fluid from getting inside the pump and/or motor, and causing contamination and mold growth. This protects both mother and baby, and the pump. A wet filter may need several hours to dry, or may need to be replaced.

For healthy, full-term babies the pump parts are:

» Washed in hot, soapy water.

» Rinsed in hot water.

» Laid out to air dry on a clean towel.

» Covered with another clean towel.

In addition:

» A bottle brush may be used on the milk-storage containers.

» NEVER use a nipple brush on the valves/membranes.

» Be gentle with this part. They often have thin edges that are easily torn, frayed, or otherwise damaged by sharp objects, including finger-nails. Swish tubular (duckbill) valves in soapy water, and gently rub flat-valve membranes with the fingertips, like cleaning a contact lens.

» NEVER put the valves/membranes on pegs (like on a bottle/nipple drying rack) to air dry.

» The valves or membranes are sensitive pieces, and poking things in or through them can warp or tear them.

» Vulnerable (preterm, small for gestational age, ill) babies may require that the pump parts be sterilized in addition to washing.

Sterilizing Pump Parts

» Start the water boiling first without placing anything else in the pot. Put sufficient water in the pot to allow the pump pieces to be covered by several inches of water once they are submerged.

» Once the water is boiling, lower the heat until the water is boiling softly.

» Pad the inside of the pot with a cotton dish towel, washcloth, or diaper. This will prevent the pump parts from warping or melting from touching the hot metal. The pad will also singe before the plastic, if the boiling pump parts are forgotten, and all the water boils away.

» Put the pump parts in, on top of your cotton-cloth padding, so that they are completely immersed in the boiling water.

» SET A TIMER. It needs to be a loud, repetitive alarm (new parents are often overtired and forgetful).

» When the timer alarm goes off, shut off the heat and allow the water and parts to cool off to a safe temperature.

» Use a set of tongs to remove the pump parts from the water.

» Lay them out to air dry on a clean towel.

» Cover them with a clean towel.

» Once dry, parts can be stored in gallon zipper-top plastic bags.

Common Concerns

Dishwashers

Pump parts can be cleaned in the dishwasher, but should not routinely be washed in one. Dishwashers use very harsh chemicals and very hot water, plus heat to dry, all of which will shorten the life of pump parts, especially the sensitive valves/membranes. Mothers who value convenience over money may want to use the dishwasher anyway. But those who are dependent on their pump may want to avoid using the dishwasher.

Sterilizing Bags

The use of microwave sterilizing bags can cause extra extreme wear on pump parts over time. Microwave sterilizing bags should be reserved for when a stove and pot are unavailable.

Cleaning Tubing

» If tubing becomes wet, it must be washed and dried before attaching it to the pump. Otherwise, fluid can be drawn into the motor area and cause mold growth, or contact the filter and shut down the pump. Immerse the tubing completely in clean, hot, soapy water. Run that soapy water through the tubing several times.

» Rinse by running a stream of hot, clean water through the tubing.

Drying the Tubing

» You can whip the tubing in the air like a lariat. Make sure you are holding the end with any hard plastic adapter on it, and that the free end is soft. Hold the tubing away from your body to avoid being hit.

» Roll the tubing back and forth on a table with the palms of your hands, like rolling dough for pretzels, or making snakes out of modeling clay. Rolling the tubing like this pulls the fluid out each of the ends.

» Blow out the fluid with a hair dryer or can of compressed air through a funnel made from a small piece of paper inserted into the larger end of the tubing. Some canned air has that little red tube, which can also be used on your pump tubing.

» You can use isopropyl alcohol. Put a few drops down the tubing and allow it to evaporate, along with the fluid.

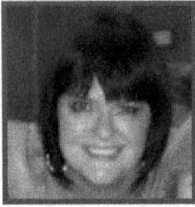

Kathleen Chiu, IBCLC, RLC. In the last 25 years, Kat has held positions as LC in a pediatrics practice, a private practice, a group LC practice, as well as both postpartum and the NICU. Kat has also worked in the breast pump industry as a lactation consultant, sales manager, product manager and a marketing resource for almost 10 years.

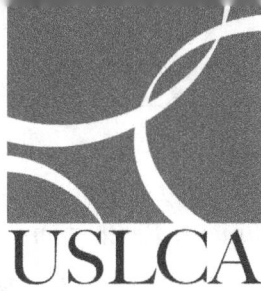

It's Not Just Milk; It's Relationship

Recent Findings in Neuroscience Show Breastfeeding's Effects Throughout the Lifespan

Kathleen Kendall-Tackett, PhD, IBCLC, RLC, FAPA[1]

Keywords: Breastfeeding, pain, depression, lactation support

The articles included in this monograph all focus on helping mothers increase and maintain their milk supplies, and emphasize the importance of human milk and its role in ensuring babies' healthy growth and development. Human milk is definitely worth all the efforts mothers put towards maintaining their supplies. As important as it is, however, we must remember one key fact when we are working with mothers: the essential element to babies' growth and development is the

---

1   kkendallt@gmail.com

mother herself. It is her responsive care that leads to secure attachment. Researchers now recognize that secure attachment forms the basis for babies' lifetime health. Breastfeeding provides both human milk and responsive care, for you cannot breastfeed without being responsive. However, in the event that a mother is not able to provide human milk for her baby, or can only bring in a partial supply, you can help her find other ways to be a responsive caregiver (such as through babywearing, infant massage, or mother-infant coaching). When working with these mothers, we must emphasize the importance of her relationship to her baby. This is the foundation for her baby's health and lifelong wellness. For those mothers who cannot bring in a full supply, or who cannot breastfeed at all, emphasizing the relationship she has with her baby might help her cope with her situation and focus on the things she can do, rather than what she cannot do.

In a 2009 article in the *Journal of the American Medical Association*, Shonkoff, Boyce, and McEwen (2009) described how early life experiences set the stage for physical health in later life. They stated that reducing *early toxic stress* was key to preventing disease in adults.

Breastfeeding is one important way to decrease early toxic stress. Recent studies have shown that breastfeeding increases babies' physical and mental well-being, and these effects go well beyond the composition of the milk. Maternal responsiveness is key to understanding these long-term effects. When mothers consistently respond to their babies' cues, they set the stage for lifelong resiliency in their offspring. And responsiveness is built into the breast-feeding relationship. We see this reflected in children's mental health. In one study of 2,900 mother–infant pairs, breastfeeding for 1 year was associated with better child mental health at every age point up to age 14 years (Oddy et al., 2009).

Breastfeeding and Maternal Depression

Maternal depression has a well-documented negative effect on babies and children. It is harmful because it impairs mothers' ability to be responsive to their babies. Depressed mothers tend to disengage from their babies and not respond to their cues. Babies experience this as highly stressful, and there can be lifelong effects from being raised by a chronically depressed mother or father (Field, Diego, & Hernandez-Reif, 2009; Kendall-Tackett, 2002, 2010; Weissman et al., 2006). Edward Tronick's still-face mother experiments are an analog of what happens with maternal depression. You can see the effects of non-response in the compelling video on page 123.

These effects are long lasting. A 20-year follow-up of children of depressed parents compared them with a matched group of adult children whose parents had no psychiatric illness. The adult children of depressed parents had three times the rate of major depression, anxiety disorders, and substance abuse compared to adult children of nondepressed parents (Weissman et al., 2006).

For many years, feeding method was not included in studies of maternal depression. In fact, for years, professionals who specialized in perinatal mental health believed that breastfeeding was a risk factor for postpartum depression. Fortunately, we now have evidence that indicates that exclusively breastfeeding mothers are at lower risk for depression. Indeed, breastfeeding protects maternal mental health (Dennis & McQueen, 2009; Groer & Davis, 2006; Kendall-Tackett, Cong, & Hale, 2011).

One reason why breastfeeding lowers depression risk is its impact on sleep. On every parameter of sleep, exclusively breastfeeding mothers fare better than their mixed- or formula-feeding counterparts: total length of sleep, minutes to get to sleep, percentage of slow-wave sleep, daytime fatigue, and perceived physical health (Blyton, Sullivan, & Edwards, 2002; Doan, Gardiner, Gay, & Lee, 2007; Kendall-Tackett et al., 2011).

Our study of 6,410 mothers indicated that exclusively breastfeeding mothers were significantly better on every sleep measure compared to their mixed- and formula-feeding counterparts. Surprisingly, there was no significant difference between the mixed- and formula-feeding mothers (Kendall-Tackett et al., 2011). In other words, exclusive breastfeeding is a different physiological experience than mixed feeding. When mothers supplement, they appear to lose the physiological benefit of breastfeeding on their sleep.

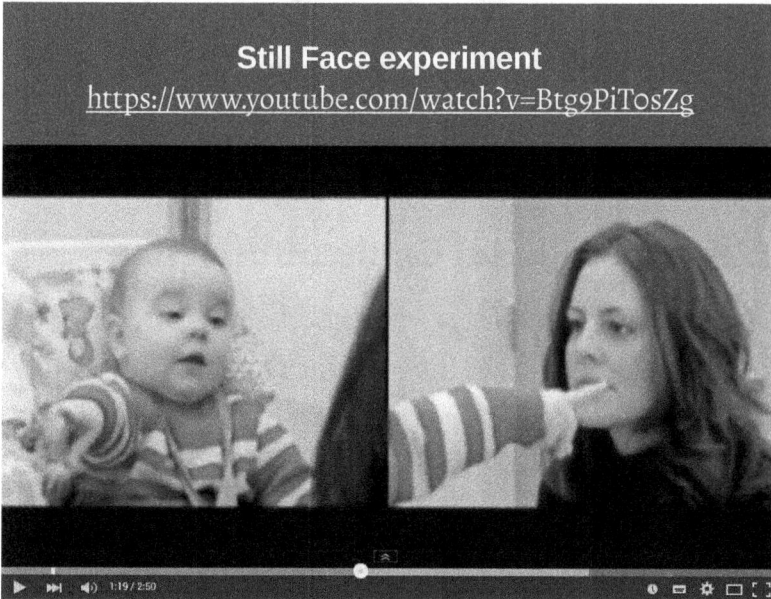

Still Face experiment
https://www.youtube.com/watch?v=Btg9PiTosZg

One study also found that breastfeeding protects babies when their mothers are depressed. This study compared four groups of mothers: mothers who were either depressed (breastfeeding or formula feeding) or nondepressed (breastfeeding or formula feeding). The measure was the babies' electroencephalogram (EEG) patterns (abnormal patterns were a symptom of depression in the infants).

The babies of depressed, breastfeeding mothers had normal EEG patterns compared to the babies of depressed, formula-feeding mothers (Jones, McFall, & Diego, 2004). *In other words, breastfeeding protected the babies from the harmful effects of their mothers' depression.* The reason for this finding comes down to maternal responsivity. The researchers discovered that the depressed, breastfeeding mothers did not disengage from their babies. They couldn't. The breast-feeding mothers looked at, touched, and made eye contact with their babies more than the mothers who were not breastfeeding. And that was enough to make a difference.

Intergenerational Cycle of Violence

Mothers with a history of childhood abuse often feel as though they do not have the tools they need to successfully parent their own children. They may wonder whether they will perpetuate the cycle of violence. Impaired sleep can be an important trigger to the intergenerational transmission of abuse. Babies of mothers with depression or posttraumatic stress disorder (PTSD) are more likely to have sleep difficulties, possibly because of mothers' elevated stress hormone levels that the babies were exposed to in utero (Field, Diego, & Hernandez-Reif, 2006; Field et al., 2007). And a recent study found that for women with PTSD and a history of childhood abuse, infant sleep difficulties and maternal depression impaired mother–infant bonding and increased the risk of intergenerational transmission of trauma (Hairston et al., 2011).

That is, of course, unless the mother breastfeeds. In Strathearn, Mamun, Najman, and O'Callaghan's (2009) 15-year longitudinal study of 7,223 Australian mother–infant pairs, breastfeeding substantially lowered the risk of maternal-perpetrated child maltreatment. Nonbreastfeeding mothers were 2.6 times more likely to be physically abusive and 3.8 times more likely to neglect their children compared to breastfeeding mothers.

The results of our recent study may help explain why this is so. In our sample of 6,410 new mothers, 994 women reported previous sexual assault. As predicted, sexual assault had a pervasive, negative effect on mothers' sleep, physical well-being, and mental health. The sexually assaulted mothers' sleep was poor, they were more tired, they were more anxious and angry, and they had more depression. But when we added feeding method to our analyses, we found that breastfeeding attenuated the effects of sexual assault and downregulated the stress response. This effect was only for exclusively breastfeeding women (Kendall-Tackett, Cong, & Hale, 2013). Anger, in particular, was lessened, and this might explain Strathearn and colleagues' (2009) findings cited earlier. Also, lower rates of depression improve maternal responsiveness, which is protective.

Attachment and Long-Term Health

We can also examine the impact of security of mother–infant attachment and its effects on long-term health. In an article written shortly before the end of their lives, attachment pioneers Ainsworth and Bowlby (1991) noted that maternal (or caregiver) responsivity was key to creating a secure attachment in infants. Ainsworth developed the primary measure of attachment in infants: the Strange Situation.

The Strange Situation has been used in thousands of studies all over the world. Secure attachment on this measure is a great predictor of child mental and physical health. And responsiveness is key. When babies are not responded to consistently, they develop insecure attachments, and these have long-term implications for health, as a recent 32-year longitudinal study of 163 people found (Puig, Englund, Simpson, & Collins, 2013).

Participants in this study were followed from birth to age 32 years. At 12 to 18 months of age, they were assessed via the Strange Situation. Those with insecure attachments had significantly more inflammation-based illnesses at age 32 years than those who had secure attachments.

These findings are likely because of the chronic activation of the inflammatory response system in those with insecure attachments.

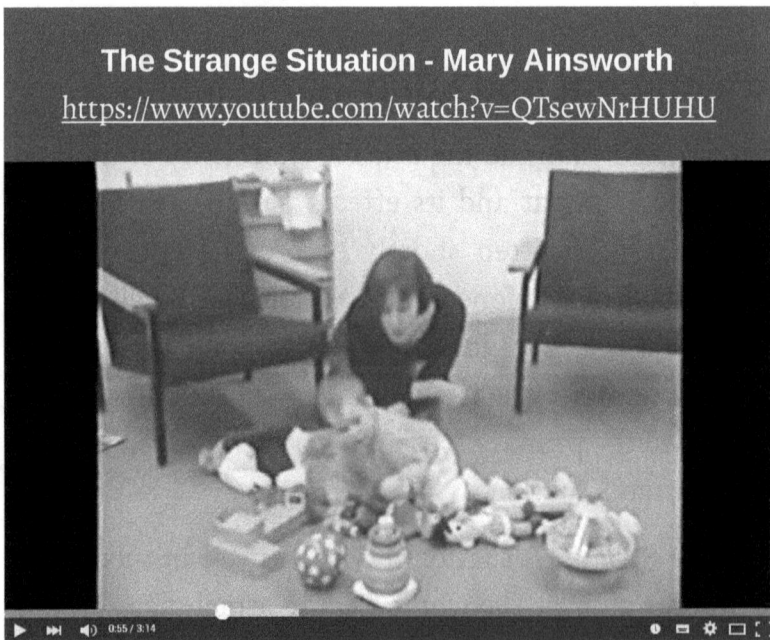

The Strange Situation - Mary Ainsworth
https://www.youtube.com/watch?v=QTsewNrHUHU

Summary

The results from these recent studies demonstrate that breastfeeding has a much larger role to play in maintaining physical and mental health than we have previously believed. It's not just the milk. Because breastfeeding increases maternal responsivity, it makes the day-to-day experience of mothering more tolerable. It increases the chances that the babies will be securely attached. And even if a mother is not able to breastfeed, being responsive to her baby will still lead to a secure attachment, which will benefit her baby's lifetime health.

Breastfeeding is so much more than just a method of feeding. It's a way of caring for a baby that will provide a lifetime's worth of good health because it provides a way for mothers to connect with their babies—even if they did not experience that kind of care themselves. In short, breastfeeding can make the world a happier and healthier place, one mother and baby at a time.

References

Ainsworth, M. D. S., & Bowlby, J. (1991). An ethological approach to personality development. *American Psychologist, 46,* 333–341.

Blyton, D. M., Sullivan, C. E., & Edwards, N. (2002). Lactation is associated with an increase in slow-wave sleep in women. *Journal of Sleep Research, 11*(4), 297–303.

Dennis, C. L., & McQueen, K. (2009). The relationship between infant-feeding outcomes and postpartum depression: A qualitative systematic review. *Pediatrics, 123,* e736–e751.

Doan, T., Gardiner, A., Gay, C. L., & Lee, K. A. (2007). Breastfeeding increases sleep duration of new parents. *Journal of Perinatal & Neonatal Nursing, 21*(3), 200–206.

Field, T., Diego, M., & Hernandez-Reif, M. (2006). Prenatal depression effects on the fetus and newborn: A review. *Infant Behavior & Development, 29*, 445–455.

Field, T., Diego, M., & Hernandez-Reif, M. (2009). Infants of depressed mothers are less responsive to faces and voices: A review. *Infant Behavior & Development, 32*(3), 239–244.

Field, T., Diego, M., Hernandez-Reif, M., Figueiredo, B., Schanberg, S., & Kuhn, C. (2007). Sleep disturbance in depressed pregnant women and their newborns. *Infant Behavior & Development, 30*, 127–133.

Groer, M. W., & Davis, M. W. (2006). Cytokines, infections, stress, and dysphoric moods in breastfeeders and formula feeders. *Journal of Obstetric, Gynecologic, and Neonatal Nursing, 35*, 599–607.

Hairston, I. S., Waxler, E., Seng, J. S., Fezzey, A. G., Rosenblum, K. L., & Muzik, M. (2011). The role of infant sleep in intergenerational transmission of trauma. *Sleep, 34*(10), 1373–1383.

Jones, N. A., McFall, B. A., & Diego, M. A. (2004). Patterns of brain electrical activity in infants of depressed mothers who breastfeed and bottle feed: The mediating role of infant temperament. *Biological Psychology, 67*, 103–124.

Kendall-Tackett, K. A. (2002). Depression in new mothers: Why it matters to the child maltreatment field. *Section on Child Maltreatment Newsletter: Division 37, American Psychological Association, 6*, 8–9.

Kendall-Tackett, K. A. (2010). *Depression in new mothers: Causes, consequences, and treatment options* (2nd ed.). London, United Kingdom: Routledge.

Kendall-Tackett, K. A., Cong, Z., & Hale, T. W. (2011). The effect of feeding method on sleep duration, maternal wellbeing, and postpartum depression. *Clinical Lactation, 2*(2), 22–26.

Kendall-Tackett, K. A., Cong, Z., & Hale, T. W. (2013). Depression, sleep quality, and maternal well-being in postpartum women with a history of sexual assault: A comparison of breastfeeding, mixed-feeding, and formula-feeding mothers. *Breastfeeding Medicine, 8*(1), 16–22.

Oddy, W. H., Kendall, G. E., Li, J., Jacoby, P., Robinson, M., de Klerk, N. H., . . . Stanley, F. J. (2009). The long-term effects of breastfeeding on child and adolescent mental health: A pregnancy cohort study followed for 14 years. *Journal of Pediatrics, 156*(4), 568–574.

Puig, J., Englund, M. M., Simpson, J. A., & Collins, W. A. (2013). Predicting adult physical illness from infant attachment: A prospective longitudinal study. *Health Psychology, 32*(4), 409–417.

Shonkoff, J. P., Boyce, W. T., & McEwen, B. S. (2009). Neuroscience, molecular biology, and the childhood roots of health disparities: Building a new framework for health promotion and disease prevention. *The Journal of the American Medical Association, 301*(21), 2252–2259. http://dx.doi.org/10.1001/jama.2009.754

Strathearn, L., Mamun, A. A., Najman, J. M., & O'Callaghan, M. J. (2009). Does breastfeeding protect against substantiated child abuse and neglect? A 15-year cohort study. *Pediatrics, 123*(2), 483–493. http://dx.doi.org/10.1542/peds.2007-3546

Weissman, M. M., Wickramaratne, P., Nomura, Y., Warner, V., Pilowsky, D., & Verdeli, H. (2006). Offspring of depressed parents: 20 years later. *American Journal of Psychiatry, 163*, 1001–1008.

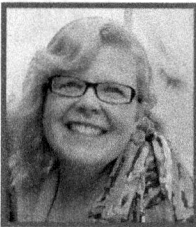

Kathleen Kendall-Tackett , PhD, IBCLC, RLC, FAPA, is a health psychologist, International Board Certified Lactation Consultant, and the owner and editor-in-chief of *Praeclarus Press*, a small press specializing in women's health.

Dr. Kendall-Tackett is editor-in-chief of *Clinical Lactation*, fellow of the American Psychological Association (APA) in Health and Trauma Psychology, past-president of the APA Division of Trauma Psychology, and editor-in-chief of *Psychological Trauma*.

Dr. Kendall-Tackett has won several awards for her work including the 2011 John Kennell and Marshall Klaus Award for Excellence in Research from DONA International (with corecipient Tom Hale). She has authored more than 390 articles or chapters and is the author or editor of 25 books on maternal depression, family violence, and breastfeeding, including *Psychology of Trauma 101* (2015) and *The Science of Mother-Infant Sleep* (2014).

Her websites are
http://www.uppitysciencechick.com,
http://www.breastfeedingmadesimple.com,
http://www.kathleenkendall-tackett.com, and
http://www.praeclaruspress.com.

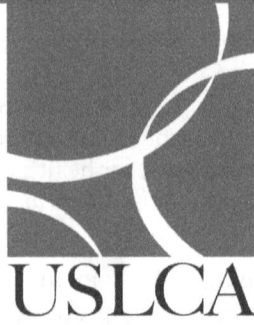

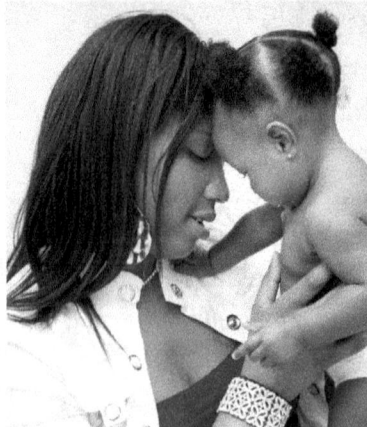

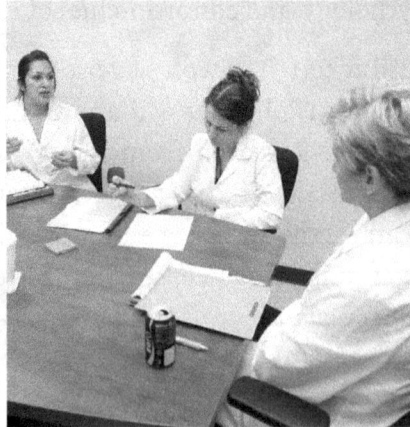

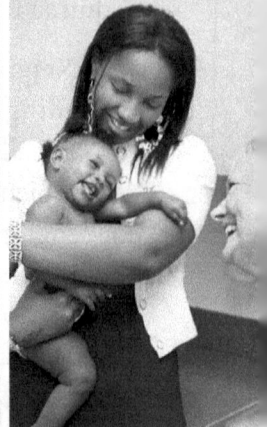

The U.S. Lactation Consultant Association Presents
Clinical Lactation Monographs

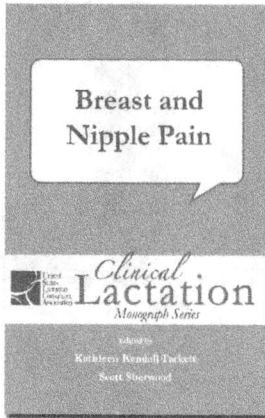

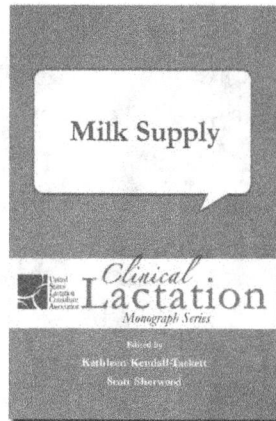

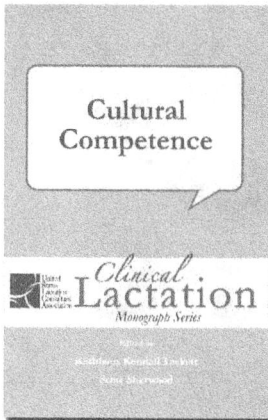

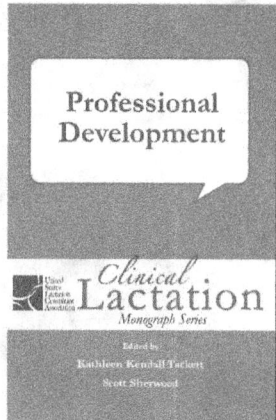

Praeclarus Press
Excellence in Women's Health

www.PraeclarusPress.com

Breastfeeding Titles from Praeclarus Press

Praeclarus Press
Excellence in Women's Health

www.PraeclarusPress.com

www.ingramcontent.com/pod-product-compliance
Lightning Source LLC
Chambersburg PA
CBHW060909280326
41934CB00007B/1250